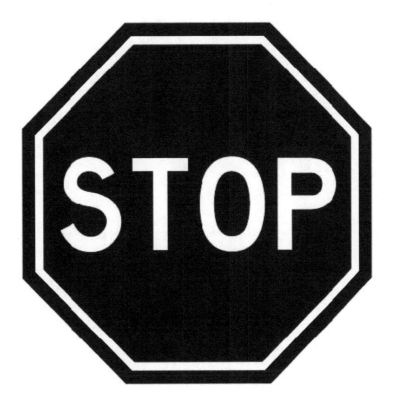

FREE Test Taking Tips DVD Offer

To help us better serve you, we have developed a Test Taking Tips DVD that we would like to give you for FREE. **This DVD covers world-class test taking tips that you can use to be even more successful when you are taking your test.**

All that we ask is that you email us your feedback about your study guide. Please let us know what you thought about it – whether that is good, bad or indifferent.

To get your **FREE Test Taking Tips DVD**, email freedvd@studyguideteam.com with "FREE DVD" in the subject line and the following information in the body of the email:

    a. The title of your study guide.

    b. Your product rating on a scale of 1-5, with 5 being the highest rating.

    c. Your feedback about the study guide. What did you think of it?

    d. Your full name and shipping address to send your free DVD.

If you have any questions or concerns, please don't hesitate to contact us at freedvd@studyguideteam.com.

Thanks again!

HESI A2 Study Guide 2019 & 2020

HESI Admission Assessment Exam Review 2019-2020
4th Edition & Practice Test Questions

Test Prep Books

Table of Contents

Quick Overview

As you draw closer to taking your exam, effective preparation becomes more and more important. Thankfully, you have this study guide to help you get ready. Use this guide to help keep your studying on track and refer to it often.

This study guide contains several key sections that will help you be successful on your exam. The guide contains tips for what you should do the night before and the day of the test. Also included are test-taking tips. Knowing the right information is not always enough. Many well-prepared test takers struggle with exams. These tips will help equip you to accurately read, assess, and answer test questions.

A large part of the guide is devoted to showing you what content to expect on the exam and to helping you better understand that content. In this guide are practice test questions so that you can see how well you have grasped the content. Then, answer explanations are provided so that you can understand why you missed certain questions.

Don't try to cram the night before you take your exam. This is not a wise strategy for a few reasons. First, your retention of the information will be low. Your time would be better used by reviewing information you already know rather than trying to learn a lot of new information. Second, you will likely become stressed as you try to gain a large amount of knowledge in a short amount of time. Third, you will be depriving yourself of sleep. So be sure to go to bed at a reasonable time the night before. Being well-rested helps you focus and remain calm.

Be sure to eat a substantial breakfast the morning of the exam. If you are taking the exam in the afternoon, be sure to have a good lunch as well. Being hungry is distracting and can make it difficult to focus. You have hopefully spent lots of time preparing for the exam. Don't let an empty stomach get in the way of success!

When travelling to the testing center, leave earlier than needed. That way, you have a buffer in case you experience any delays. This will help you remain calm and will keep you from missing your appointment time at the testing center.

Be sure to pace yourself during the exam. Don't try to rush through the exam. There is no need to risk performing poorly on the exam just so you can leave the testing center early. Allow yourself to use all of the allotted time if needed.

Remain positive while taking the exam even if you feel like you are performing poorly. Thinking about the content you should have mastered will not help you perform better on the exam.

Once the exam is complete, take some time to relax. Even if you feel that you need to take the exam again, you will be well served by some down time before you begin studying again. It's often easier to convince yourself to study if you know that it will come with a reward!

Test-Taking Strategies

1. Predicting the Answer

When you feel confident in your preparation for a multiple-choice test, try predicting the answer before reading the answer choices. This is especially useful on questions that test objective factual knowledge. By predicting the answer before reading the available choices, you eliminate the possibility that you will be distracted or led astray by an incorrect answer choice. You will feel more confident in your selection if you read the question, predict the answer, and then find your prediction among the answer choices. After using this strategy, be sure to still read all of the answer choices carefully and completely. If you feel unprepared, you should not attempt to predict the answers. This would be a waste of time and an opportunity for your mind to wander in the wrong direction.

2. Reading the Whole Question

Too often, test takers scan a multiple-choice question, recognize a few familiar words, and immediately jump to the answer choices. Test authors are aware of this common impatience, and they will sometimes prey upon it. For instance, a test author might subtly turn the question into a negative, or he or she might redirect the focus of the question right at the end. The only way to avoid falling into these traps is to read the entirety of the question carefully before reading the answer choices.

3. Looking for Wrong Answers

Long and complicated multiple-choice questions can be intimidating. One way to simplify a difficult multiple-choice question is to eliminate all of the answer choices that are clearly wrong. In most sets of answers, there will be at least one selection that can be dismissed right away. If the test is administered on paper, the test taker could draw a line through it to indicate that it may be ignored; otherwise, the test taker will have to perform this operation mentally or on scratch paper. In either case, once the obviously incorrect answers have been eliminated, the remaining choices may be considered. Sometimes identifying the clearly wrong answers will give the test taker some information about the correct answer. For instance, if one of the remaining answer choices is a direct opposite of one of the eliminated answer choices, it may well be the correct answer. The opposite of obviously wrong is obviously right! Of course, this is not always the case. Some answers are obviously incorrect simply because they are irrelevant to the question being asked. Still, identifying and eliminating some incorrect answer choices is a good way to simplify a multiple-choice question.

4. Don't Overanalyze

Anxious test takers often overanalyze questions. When you are nervous, your brain will often run wild, causing you to make associations and discover clues that don't actually exist. If you feel that this may be a problem for you, do whatever you can to slow down during the test. Try taking a deep breath or counting to ten. As you read and consider the question, restrict yourself to the particular words used by the author. Avoid thought tangents about what the author *really* meant, or what he or she was *trying* to say. The only things that matter on a multiple-choice test are the words that are actually in the question. You must avoid reading too much into a multiple-choice question, or supposing that the writer meant something other than what he or she wrote.

5. No Need for Panic

It is wise to learn as many strategies as possible before taking a multiple-choice test, but it is likely that you will come across a few questions for which you simply don't know the answer. In this situation, avoid panicking. Because most multiple-choice tests include dozens of questions, the relative value of a single wrong answer is small. As much as possible, you should compartmentalize each question on a multiple-choice test. In other words, you should not allow your feelings about one question to affect your success on the others. When you find a question that you either don't understand or don't know how to answer, just take a deep breath and do your best. Read the entire question slowly and carefully. Try rephrasing the question a couple of different ways. Then, read all of the answer choices carefully. After eliminating obviously wrong answers, make a selection and move on to the next question.

6. Confusing Answer Choices

When working on a difficult multiple-choice question, there may be a tendency to focus on the answer choices that are the easiest to understand. Many people, whether consciously or not, gravitate to the answer choices that require the least concentration, knowledge, and memory. This is a mistake. When you come across an answer choice that is confusing, you should give it extra attention. A question might be confusing because you do not know the subject matter to which it refers. If this is the case, don't eliminate the answer before you have affirmatively settled on another. When you come across an answer choice of this type, set it aside as you look at the remaining choices. If you can confidently assert that one of the other choices is correct, you can leave the confusing answer aside. Otherwise, you will need to take a moment to try to better understand the confusing answer choice. Rephrasing is one way to tease out the sense of a confusing answer choice.

7. Your First Instinct

Many people struggle with multiple-choice tests because they overthink the questions. If you have studied sufficiently for the test, you should be prepared to trust your first instinct once you have carefully and completely read the question and all of the answer choices. There is a great deal of research suggesting that the mind can come to the correct conclusion very quickly once it has obtained all of the relevant information. At times, it may seem to you as if your intuition is working faster even than your reasoning mind. This may in fact be true. The knowledge you obtain while studying may be retrieved from your subconscious before you have a chance to work out the associations that support it. Verify your instinct by working out the reasons that it should be trusted.

8. Key Words

Many test takers struggle with multiple-choice questions because they have poor reading comprehension skills. Quickly reading and understanding a multiple-choice question requires a mixture of skill and experience. To help with this, try jotting down a few key words and phrases on a piece of scrap paper. Doing this concentrates the process of reading and forces the mind to weigh the relative importance of the question's parts. In selecting words and phrases to write down, the test taker thinks about the question more deeply and carefully. This is especially true for multiple-choice questions that are preceded by a long prompt.

9. Subtle Negatives

One of the oldest tricks in the multiple-choice test writer's book is to subtly reverse the meaning of a question with a word like *not* or *except*. If you are not paying attention to each word in the question, you can easily be led astray by this trick. For instance, a common question format is, "Which of the following is…?" Obviously, if the question instead is, "Which of the following is not…?," then the answer will be quite different. Even worse, the test makers are aware of the potential for this mistake and will include one answer choice that would be correct if the question were not negated or reversed. A test taker who misses the reversal will find what he or she believes to be a correct answer and will be so confident that he or she will fail to reread the question and discover the original error. The only way to avoid this is to practice a wide variety of multiple-choice questions and to pay close attention to each and every word.

10. Reading Every Answer Choice

It may seem obvious, but you should always read every one of the answer choices! Too many test takers fall into the habit of scanning the question and assuming that they understand the question because they recognize a few key words. From there, they pick the first answer choice that answers the question they believe they have read. Test takers who read all of the answer choices might discover that one of the latter answer choices is actually *more* correct. Moreover, reading all of the answer choices can remind you of facts related to the question that can help you arrive at the correct answer. Sometimes, a misstatement or incorrect detail in one of the latter answer choices will trigger your memory of the subject and will enable you to find the right answer. Failing to read all of the answer choices is like not reading all of the items on a restaurant menu: you might miss out on the perfect choice.

11. Spot the Hedges

One of the keys to success on multiple-choice tests is paying close attention to every word. This is never truer than with words like almost, most, some, and sometimes. These words are called "hedges" because they indicate that a statement is not totally true or not true in every place and time. An absolute statement will contain no hedges, but in many subjects, the answers are not always straightforward or absolute. There are always exceptions to the rules in these subjects. For this reason, you should favor those multiple-choice questions that contain hedging language. The presence of qualifying words indicates that the author is taking special care with his or her words, which is certainly important when composing the right answer. After all, there are many ways to be wrong, but there is only one way to be right! For this reason, it is wise to avoid answers that are absolute when taking a multiple-choice test. An absolute answer is one that says things are either all one way or all another. They often include words like *every*, *always*, *best*, and *never*. If you are taking a multiple-choice test in a subject that doesn't lend itself to absolute answers, be on your guard if you see any of these words.

12. Long Answers

In many subject areas, the answers are not simple. As already mentioned, the right answer often requires hedges. Another common feature of the answers to a complex or subjective question are qualifying clauses, which are groups of words that subtly modify the meaning of the sentence. If the question or answer choice describes a rule to which there are exceptions or the subject matter is complicated, ambiguous, or confusing, the correct answer will require many words in order to be expressed clearly and accurately. In essence, you should not be deterred by answer choices that seem excessively long. Oftentimes, the author of the text will not be able to write the correct answer without offering some qualifications and modifications. Your job is to read the answer choices thoroughly and completely and to select the one that most accurately and precisely answers the question.

13. Restating to Understand

Sometimes, a question on a multiple-choice test is difficult not because of what it asks but because of how it is written. If this is the case, restate the question or answer choice in different words. This process serves a couple of important purposes. First, it forces you to concentrate on the core of the question. In order to rephrase the question accurately, you have to understand it well. Rephrasing the question will concentrate your mind on the key words and ideas. Second, it will present the information to your mind in a fresh way. This process may trigger your memory and render some useful scrap of information picked up while studying.

14. True Statements

Sometimes an answer choice will be true in itself, but it does not answer the question. This is one of the main reasons why it is essential to read the question carefully and completely before proceeding to the answer choices. Too often, test takers skip ahead to the answer choices and look for true statements. Having found one of these, they are content to select it without reference to the question above. Obviously, this provides an easy way for test makers to play tricks. The savvy test taker will always read the entire question before turning to the answer choices. Then, having settled on a correct answer choice, he or she will refer to the original question and ensure that the selected answer is relevant. The mistake of choosing a correct-but-irrelevant answer choice is especially common on questions related to specific pieces of objective knowledge. A prepared test taker will have a wealth of factual knowledge at his or her disposal, and should not be careless in its application.

15. No Patterns

One of the more dangerous ideas that circulates about multiple-choice tests is that the correct answers tend to fall into patterns. These erroneous ideas range from a belief that B and C are the most common right answers, to the idea that an unprepared test-taker should answer "A-B-A-C-A-D-A-B-A." It cannot be emphasized enough that pattern-seeking of this type is exactly the WRONG way to approach a multiple-choice test. To begin with, it is highly unlikely that the test maker will plot the correct answers according to some predetermined pattern. The questions are scrambled and delivered in a random order. Furthermore, even if the test maker was following a pattern in the assignation of correct answers, there is no reason why the test taker would know which pattern he or she was using. Any attempt to discern a pattern in the answer choices is a waste of time and a distraction from the real work of taking the test. A test taker would be much better served by extra preparation before the test than by reliance on a pattern in the answers.

FREE DVD OFFER

Don't forget that doing well on your exam includes both understanding the test content and understanding how to use what you know to do well on the test. We offer a completely FREE Test Taking Tips DVD that covers world class test taking tips that you can use to be even more successful when you are taking your test.

All that we ask is that you email us your feedback about your study guide. To get your **FREE Test Taking Tips DVD**, email freedvd@studyguideteam.com with "FREE DVD" in the subject line and the following information in the body of the email:

- The title of your study guide.
- Your product rating on a scale of 1-5, with 5 being the highest rating.
- Your feedback about the study guide. What did you think of it?
- Your full name and shipping address to send your free DVD.

Introduction to the HESI Admission Assessment Exam

Function of the Test

The Health Education Systems, Inc. (HESI) Admission Assessment (A2) Exam is an entrance exam intended for high school graduates seeking admission to post-secondary health programs such as nursing schools. Test-takers have typically not received any training in specific medical subjects. The test is offered nationwide by the colleges and universities that require it as part of an applicant's admission package.

Test Administration

Many of the specifics of the process of HESI administration are determined at the discretion of the testing institution. For instance, each school may choose to administer the entire HESI exam or any portion thereof. Accordingly, there is no set process or schedule for taking the exam; instead, the schedule is determined on a case-by-case basis by the institution administering the exam. Likewise, the cost of the HESI is set by the administering institution. The typical cost is usually around $40-$70.

Find out ahead of time which sections you will be required to take so that you can focus your studying on those areas.

Retesting is generally permitted by HESI, but individual schools may have their own rules on the subject. Likewise, individual schools may set their own policies on whether section scores from different sessions of the HESI can be combined to get one score, or whether a score must come from one coherent session. Students with disabilities may seek accommodations from the schools administering the exam.

Test Format

The exam can include up to eight academic sections with the following distribution of questions:

Section	# of Questions
Mathematics	50
Reading Comprehension	55
Vocabulary	50
Grammar	50
Biology	25
Chemistry	25
Anatomy & Physiology	25
Physics	25

Additionally, there is a Personality Profile and Learning Style Assessment that may be included. Like the academic sections, schools can pick and choose whether to include one, both, or neither of these assessments. Each takes about 15 minutes, and you do not need to study for them.

Scoring

Prospective students and their educational institutions both receive detailed score reports after a prospective applicant completes the exam. Individual student reports include scoring explanations and breakdowns by topic for incorrect answers. The test taker's results can also include study tips based on the individual's Learning Style assessment and identification of the test taker's dominant personality type, strengths, weaknesses, and suggested learning techniques, based on the Personality Profile.

There is no set passing score for the HESI. Instead, individual schools set their own requirements and processes for incorporating scores into admissions decisions. However, HESI recommends that RN and HP programs require a 75% score to pass, and that LPN/LVN programs require a 70% score to pass.

Mathematics

Numbers usually serve as an adjective representing a quantity of objects. They function as placeholders for a value. Numbers can be better understood by their type and related characteristics.

Definitions

A few definitions:

Whole numbers: describes a set of numbers that does not contain any fractions or decimals. The set of whole numbers includes zero.

> Example: 0, 1, 2, 3, 4, 189, 293 are all whole numbers.

Integers: describes whole numbers and their negative counterparts. (Zero does not have a negative counterpart here. Instead, zero is its own negative.)

> Example: -1, -2, -3, -4, -5, 0, 1, 2, 3, 4, 5 are all integers.

-1, -2, -3, -4, -5 are considered negative integers and 1, 2, 3, 4, 5 are considered positive integers.

Absolute value: describes the value of a number regardless of its sign. The symbol for absolute value is | |.

> Example: The absolute value of 24 is 24 or $|24| = 24$.

The absolute value of -693 is 693 or $|-693| = 693$.

Even numbers: describes any number that can be divided by 2 evenly, meaning the answer has no decimal or remainder portion.

> Example: 2, 4, 9082, -2, -16, -504 are all considered even numbers, because they can be divided by 2, without a remainder or decimal. It does not matter whether the number is positive or negative.

Odd numbers: describes any number that does not divide evenly by 2.

> Example: 1, 21, 541, 3003, -9, -63, -1257 are all considered odd numbers, because they cannot be divided by 2 without a remainder or a decimal.

Prime numbers: describes a number that is only evenly divisible, resulting in no remainder or decimal, by 1 and itself.

> Example: 2, 3, 7, 13, 113 are all considered prime numbers, because they can only be evenly divided by 1 and itself.

Composite numbers: describes a positive integer that is formed by multiplying two smaller integers together. Composite numbers can be divided evenly by numbers other than 1 or itself.

> Example: 24, 66, 2348, 10002 are all considered composite numbers, because they are the result of multiplying two smaller integers together. In particular, these are all divisible by 2.

Decimals: designated by a decimal point which indicates that what follows the point is a value that is less than 1 and is added to the integer number preceding the decimal point. The digit immediately following the decimal point is in the tenths place, the digit following the tenths place is in the hundredths place, and so on.

For example, the decimal number 1.735 has a value greater than 1 but less than 2. The 7 represents seven tenths of the unit 1 (0.7 or $\frac{7}{10}$); the 3 represents three hundredths of 1 (0.03 or $\frac{3}{100}$); and the 5 represents five thousandths of 1 (0.005 or $\frac{5}{1000}$).

Real numbers: describes rational numbers and irrational numbers.

Rational numbers: describes any number that can be expressed as a fraction, with a non-zero denominator. Since any integer can be written with 1 in the denominator without changing its value, all integers are considered rational numbers. Every rational number has a decimal expression that terminates or repeats. That is, any rational number either will have a countable number of nonzero digits or will end with an ellipses or a bar (3.6666... or $3.\bar{6}$) to depict repeating decimal digits. Some examples of rational numbers include 12, -3.54, $110.\overline{256}$, $\frac{-35}{10}$, and $4.\bar{7}$.

Irrational numbers: describes numbers which cannot be written as a finite decimal. Pi (π) is considered to be an irrational number because its decimal portion is unending or a non-repeating decimal. The most common irrational number is π, which has an endless and non-repeating decimal, but there are other well-known irrational numbers like e and $\sqrt{2}$.

Basic Addition and Subtraction

Addition
Addition is the combination of two numbers so their quantities are added together cumulatively. The sign for an addition operation is the + symbol. For example, 9 + 6 = 15. The 9 and 6 combine to achieve a cumulative value, called a **sum**.

Addition holds the **commutative property**, which means that numbers in an addition equation can be switched without altering the result. The formula for the commutative property is a + b = b + a. Let's look at a few examples to see how the commutative property works:

$$7 = 3 + 4 = 4 + 3 = 7$$

$$20 = 12 + 8 = 8 + 12 = 20$$

Addition also holds the **associative property**, which means that the grouping of numbers doesn't matter in an addition problem. In other words, the presence or absence of parentheses is irrelevant. The formula for the associative property is (a + b) + c = a + (b + c). Here are some examples of the associative property at work:

$$30 = (6 + 14) + 10 = 6 + (14 + 10) = 30$$

$$35 = 8 + (2 + 25) = (8 + 2) + 25 = 35$$

There are set columns for addition: ones, tens, hundreds, thousands, ten-thousands, hundred-thousands, millions, and so on. To add how many units there are total, each column needs to be combined, starting from the right, or the ones column.

THOUSANDS	HUNDREDS	TENS	ONES

Every 10 units in the ones column equals one in the tens column, and every 10 units in the tens column equals one in the hundreds column, and so on.

Example: The number 5432 has 2 ones, 3 tens, 4 hundreds, and 5 thousands. The number 371 has 3 hundreds, 7 tens and 1 one. To combine, or add, these two numbers, simply add up how many units of each column exist. The best way to do this is by lining up the columns:

$$
\begin{array}{r}
5\ 4\ 3\ 2 \\
+\quad 3\ 7\ 1 \\
\hline
\end{array}
$$

The ones column adds 2 + 1 for a total (sum) of 3.

The tens column adds 3 + 7 for a total of 10; since 10 of that unit was collected, add 1 to the hundreds column to denote the total in the next column:

$$
\begin{array}{r}
1\quad\quad \\
5\ 4\ 3\ 2 \\
+\quad 3\ 7\ 1 \\
\hline
0\ 3
\end{array}
$$

When adding the hundreds column this extra 1 needs to be combined, so it would be the sum of 4, 3, and 1.

$$4 + 3 + 1 = 8$$

The last, or thousands, column listed would be the sum of 5. Since there are no other numbers in this column, that is the final total.

The answer would look as follows:

$$
\begin{array}{r}
5\ 4\ 3\ 2 \\
+\quad 3\ 7\ 1 \\
\hline
5\ 8\ 0\ 3
\end{array}
$$

Example
Find the sum of 9,734 and 895.

Set up the problem:

$$
\begin{array}{r}
9\ 7\ 3\ 4 \\
+\quad 8\ 9\ 5 \\
\hline
\end{array}
$$

Total the columns:

$$
\begin{array}{r}
9\ 7\ 3\ 4 \\
+\quad 8\ 9\ 5 \\
\hline
1\ 0\ 6\ 2\ 9
\end{array}
$$

In this example, another column (ten-thousands) is added to the left of the thousands column, to denote a carryover of 10 units in the thousands column. The final sum is 10,629.

When adding using all negative integers, the total is negative. The integers are simply added together and the negative symbol is tacked on.

$$(-12) + (-435) = -447$$

Subtraction

Subtraction is taking away one number from another, so their quantities are reduced. The sign designating a subtraction operation is the – symbol, and the result is called the **difference**. For example, 9 - 6 = 3. The number *6* detracts from the number *9* to reach the difference *3*.

Unlike addition, subtraction follows neither the commutative nor associative properties. The order and grouping in subtraction impact the result.

$$15 = 22 - 7 \neq 7 - 22 = -15$$

$$3 = (10 - 5) - 2 \neq 10 - (5 - 2) = 7$$

When working through subtraction problems involving larger numbers, it's necessary to regroup the numbers. Let's work through a practice problem using regrouping:

$$
\begin{array}{r}
3\ 2\ 5 \\
-\ \ 7\ 7 \\
\hline
\end{array}
$$

Here, it is clear that the ones and tens columns for 77 are greater than the ones and tens columns for 325. To subtract this number, borrow from the tens and hundreds columns. When borrowing from a column, subtracting 1 from the lender column will add 10 to the borrower column:

$$
\begin{array}{r}
{}^{3\text{-}1}\ \ {}^{10+2\text{-}1}\ \ {}^{10+5} \\
-\quad\quad 7\quad\quad 7
\end{array}
\ = \
\begin{array}{r}
2\ \ \ 11\ \ 15 \\
-\quad\ \ 7\ \ \ 7 \\
\hline
2\ \ \ 4\ \ \ 8
\end{array}
$$

After ensuring that each digit in the top row is greater than the digit in the corresponding bottom row, subtraction can proceed as normal, and the answer is found to be 248.

<u>Addition and Subtraction with Negative Integers</u>
When adding mixed-sign integers, determine which integer has the larger absolute value. Absolute value is the distance of a number from zero on the number line. Absolute value is indicated by these symbols: | |.

Take this equation for example:

$$12 + (-435)$$

The absolute value of each of the numbers is as follows:

$$|12| = 12$$

$$|-435| = 435$$

Since -435 is the larger integer, the final number will have its sign. In this case, that sign is negative. Now, subtract the smaller integer from the larger one. If you work out the equation, it will look like this:

$$12 + (-435) = -423$$

Mathematically, the equation looks like the one above, but practically speaking you will be doing it like this:

$$435 - 12 = 423$$

(then add the negative sign)

When using subtraction with negative integers, every unmarked integer is assumed to have a positive sign unless it is clearly marked as a negative integer. Subtracting an integer is the same as adding a negative integer.

<u>Example:</u>
-3 - 4
-3 + (-4)
-3 + (-4) = -7

Subtracting a negative integer is the same as adding a positive integer.

<u>Example</u>
-3 - (-4)
-3 + 4
-3 + 4 = 1

Multiplication of Whole Numbers

Multiplication involves adding together multiple copies of a number. It is indicated by an × symbol or a number immediately outside of a parenthesis. For example:

$$5(8 - 2)$$

The two numbers being multiplied together are called **factors**, and their result is called a **product**. For example, $9 \times 6 = 54$. This can be shown alternatively by expansion of either the 9 or the 6:

$$9 \times 6 = 9 + 9 + 9 + 9 + 9 + 9 = 54$$

$$9 \times 6 = 6 + 6 + 6 + 6 + 6 + 6 + 6 + 6 + 6 = 54$$

Like addition, multiplication holds the commutative and associative properties:

$$115 = 23 \times 5 = 5 \times 23 = 115$$

$$84 = 3 \times (7 \times 4) = (3 \times 7) \times 4 = 84$$

Multiplication also follows the **distributive property**, which allows the multiplication to be distributed through parentheses. The formula for distribution is $a \times (b + c) = ab + ac$. This is clear after the examples:

$$45 = 5 \times 9 = 5(3 + 6) = (5 \times 3) + (5 \times 6) = 15 + 30 = 45$$

$$20 = 4 \times 5 = 4(10 - 5) = (4 \times 10) - (4 \times 5) = 40 - 20 = 20$$

For larger-number multiplication, how the numbers are lined up can ease the process. It is simplest to put the number with the most digits on top and the number with fewer digits on the bottom. If they have the same number of digits, select one for the top and one for the bottom. Line up the problem, and begin by multiplying the far right column on the top and the far right column on the bottom. If the answer to a column is more than 9, the ones place digit will be written below that column and the tens place digit will carry to the top of the next column to be added after those digits are multiplied. Write the answer below that column. Move to the next column to the left on the top, and multiply it by the same far right column on the bottom. Keep moving to the left one column at a time on the top number until the end.

Example
Multiply 37×8

Line up the numbers, placing the one with the most digits on top.

$$
\begin{array}{r}
3\ 7 \\
\times \quad 8 \\
\hline
\end{array}
$$

Multiply the far right column on the top with the far right column on the bottom (7 x 8). Write the answer, 56, as below: The ones value, 6, gets recorded, the tens value, 5, is carried.

$$
\begin{array}{r}
{\scriptstyle +5} \\
3\ 7 \\
\text{X} \quad 8 \\
\hline
6
\end{array}
$$

Move to the next column left on the top number and multiply with the far right bottom (3 x 8). Remember to add any carry over after multiplying: 3 x 8 = 24, 24 + 5 = 29. Since there are no more digits on top, write the entire number below.

$$
\begin{array}{r}
{\scriptstyle +5} \\
3\ 7 \\
\text{X} \quad 8 \\
\hline
2\ 9\ 6
\end{array}
$$

The solution is 296

If there is more than one column to the bottom number, move to the row below the first strand of answers, mark a zero in the far right column, and then begin the multiplication process again with the far right column on top and the second column from the right on the bottom. For each digit in the bottom number, there will be a row of answers, each padded with the respective number of zeros on the right. Finally, add up all of the answer rows for one total number.

Example: Multiply 512×36.

Line up the numbers (the one with the most digits on top) to multiply.

Begin with the right column on top and the right column on bottom (2×6).

$$
\begin{array}{r}
5\ 1\ 2 \\
\text{X} \quad 3\ 6 \\
\hline
\end{array}
$$

Move one column left on top and multiply by the far right column on the bottom (1×6). Add the carry over after multiplying: $1 \times 6 = 6, 6 + 1 = 7$.

$$
\begin{array}{r}
{\scriptstyle +1} \\
5\ 1\ 2 \\
\text{x} \quad 3\ 6 \\
\hline
7\ 2
\end{array}
$$

Move one column left on top and multiply by the far right column on the bottom (5×6). Since this is the last digit on top, write the whole answer below.

$$
\begin{array}{r}
5\ 1\ 2 \\
\text{X} \quad 3\ 6 \\
\hline
3\ 0\ 7\ 2
\end{array}
$$

15

Now to the second column on the bottom number. Starting on the far right column on the top, repeat this pattern for the next number left on the bottom (2 × 3). Write the answers below the first line of answers; remember to begin with a zero placeholder on the far right.

```
      5 1 2
  X     3 6
  3 0 7 2
        6 0
```

Continue the pattern (1 × 3).

```
      5 1 2
  X     3 6
  3 0 7 2
      3 6 0
```

Since this is the last digit on top, write the whole answer below.

```
      5 1 2
  x     3 6
  3 0 7 2
1 5 3 6 0
```

Now add the answer rows together. Pay attention to ensure they are aligned correctly.

```
      5 1 2
  x     3 6
  3 0 7 2
1 5 3 6 0
1 8 4 3 2
```

The solution is 18,432.

Division of Whole Numbers

Division and multiplication are inverses of each other in the same way that addition and subtraction are opposites. The signs designating a division operation are the ÷ and / symbols. In division, the second number divides into the first.

The number before the division sign is called the **dividend** or, if expressed as a fraction, the **numerator.** For example, in $a \div b$, a is the dividend, while in $\frac{a}{b}$, a is the numerator.

The number after the division sign is called the **divisor** or, if expressed as a fraction, the **denominator.** For example, in $a \div b$, b is the divisor, while in $\frac{a}{b}$, b is the denominator.

Like subtraction, division doesn't follow the commutative property, as it matters which number comes before the division sign, and division doesn't follow the associative or distributive properties for the same reason. For example:

$$\frac{3}{2} = 9 \div 6 \neq 6 \div 9 = \frac{2}{3}$$

$$2 = 10 \div 5 = (30 \div 3) \div 5 \neq 30 \div (3 \div 5) = 30 \div \frac{3}{5} = 50$$

$$25 = 20 + 5 = (40 \div 2) + (40 \div 8) \neq 40 \div (2 + 8) = 40 \div 10 = 4$$

The answer to a division problem is called the **quotient.** If a divisor doesn't divide into a dividend an integer number of times, whatever is left over is termed the **remainder.** The remainder can be further divided out into decimal form by using long division; however, this doesn't always give a quotient with a finite number of decimal places, so the remainder can also be expressed as a fraction over the original divisor.

<u>Example</u>
Divide 1050/42 or 1050 ÷ 42.

Set up the problem with the denominator being divided into the numerator.

$$4\,2\overline{\smash{)}1\,0\,5\,0}$$

Check for divisibility into the first unit of the numerator, 1.

42 cannot go into 1, so add on the next unit in the denominator, 0.

42 cannot go into 10, so add on the next unit in the denominator, 5.

42 can be divided into 105, two times. Write the 2 over the 5 in 105 and multiply 42 x 2. Write the 84 under 105 for subtraction and note the remainder, 21 is less than 42.

$$
\begin{array}{r}
2 \\
4\,2\overline{\smash{)}1\,0\,5\,0} \\
-\,8\,4 \\
\hline
2\,1
\end{array}
$$

Drop the next digit in the numerator down to the remainder (making 21 into 210) to create a number 42 can divide into. 42 divides into 210 five times. Write the 5 over the 0 and multiply 42 × 5.

$$
\begin{array}{r}
2\,5 \\
4\,2\overline{\smash{)}1\,0\,5\,0} \\
-\,8\,4 \\
\hline
2\,1\,0
\end{array}
$$

Write the 210 under 210 for subtraction. The remainder is 0.

$$
\begin{array}{r}
25 \\
4\,2\,|\overline{1\,0\,5\,0}} \\
-\,8\,4 \\
\hline
2\,1\,0 \\
-\,2\,1\,0 \\
\hline
0
\end{array}
$$

The solution is 25.

<u>Example</u>
Divide 375/4 or 375 ÷ 4.

Set up the problem.

$$4\,|\overline{3\,7\,5}}$$

4 cannot divide into 3, so add the next unit from the numerator, 7. 4 divides into 37 nine times, so write the 9 above the 7. Multiply $4 \times 9 = 36$. Write the 36 under the 37 for subtraction. The remainder is 1 (1 is less than 4).

$$
\begin{array}{r}
9 \\
4\,|\overline{3\,7\,5}} \\
-\,3\,6 \\
\hline
1
\end{array}
$$

Drop the next digit in the numerator, 5, making the remainder 15. 4 divides into 15, three times, so write the 3 above the 5. Multiply 4×3. Write the 12 under the 15 for subtraction, remainder is 3 (3 is less than 4).

$$
\begin{array}{r}
9\,3 \\
4\,|\overline{3\,7\,5}} \\
-\,3\,6 \\
\hline
1\,5 \\
-\,1\,2 \\
\hline
3
\end{array}
$$

The solution is 93 remainder 3 or 93 ¾ (the remainder can be written over the original denominator).

Decimals

Decimals mark the division between the whole portion and the fractional (or decimal) portion of a number. For example, 3.15 has 3 in the whole portion and 15 in the fractional or decimal portion. A number such as 645 is all whole, but there is still a decimal place. The decimal place in 645 is to the right of the 5, but usually not written, since there is no fractional or decimal portion to this number. The same number can be written as 645.0 or 645.00 or 645.000, etc. The position of the decimal place can change the entire value of a number, and impact a calculation. In the United States, the decimal place is used when representing money. You'll often be asked to round to a certain decimal place. Here is a review of some basic decimal **place value** names:

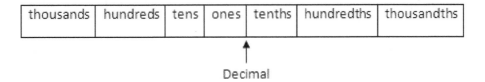

thousands	hundreds	tens	ones	tenths	hundredths	thousandths

Decimal

The number 12,302.2 would be read as "twelve thousand, three hundred two and two-tenths."

In the United States, a period denotes the decimal place; however, some countries use a comma. The comma is used in the United States to separate thousands, millions, and so on.

To round to the nearest whole number (eliminating the decimal portion), the example would become 12,302. For rounding, go to the number that is one place to the right of what you are rounding to. If the number is 0 through 4, there will be no change. For numbers 5 through 9, round up to the next whole number.

Example
Round 6,423.7 to the ones place.

Since the tenths place is the position to the right of the ones place, we use that number to determine if we round up or not. In this case, the 3 is in the ones place and the 7 is in the tenths place. (6,42_3_.7)

The 7 in the tenths place means we round the 3 up, so the final number will be 6,424.0

Example
Round 542.88 to the nearest tens

Since the ones place is the position to the right of the tens, we use that number to determine if we round up or not. In this case, the 4 is in the tens place and the 2 is in the ones place (5_42_.88).

The 2 in the ones place means we do not round the 4 up, so the final number will be 540.00

Note: Everything to the right of the rounded position goes to 0 as a placeholder.

Example: Say you wanted to post an advertisement to sell a used vehicle for $2000.00. However, when typing the price, you accidentally moved the decimal over one place to the left. Now the asking price appears as $200.00. This difference of a factor of 10 is dramatic. As numbers get bigger or smaller, the impact of this mistake becomes more pronounced. If you were looking to sell a condo for $1,000,000.00, but made an error and moved the decimal place to the left one position, the price posts at $100,000.00. A mistake of a factor of 10 cost $900,000.00.

In dividing by 10, you move the decimal one position to the left, making a smaller number than the original. If multiplying by 10, move the decimal one position to the right, making a larger number than the original.

Example
Divide 100 by 10 or 100 ÷ 10.

Move the decimal one place to the left, so the result is a smaller number than the original.

$$100 \div 10 = 10$$

Example
Divide 1.0 by 10 or 1.0 ÷ 10.

Move the decimal one place to the left, so the result is a smaller number than the original.

$$1.0 \div 10 = 0.1$$

Example
Multiply 100 by 10 or 100 x 10.

Move the decimal one place to the right, so the result is a larger number than the original.

$$100 \times 10 = 1000$$

Example
Multiply 0.1 by 10 or 0.1 x 10.

Move the decimal one place to the right, so the result is a larger number than the original.

$$0.1 \times 10 = 1.0$$

Prefixes

Moving the decimal place to the left or to the right illustrates multiplying or dividing by factors of 10. The metric system of units for measurement utilizes factors of 10 as displayed in the following table:

kilo	1000 units
hecto	100 units
deca	10 units
base unit	
deci	0.1 units
centi	0.01 units
milli	0.001 units

It is important to have the ability to quickly manipulate by 10 according to prefixes for units.

Example: How many milliliters are in 5 liters of saline solution?

There are 1000 milliliters for every 1 liter. If we have 5 liters, it would be $5 \times 1000 = 5000$ mL

You may also count the zeros and which side of the decimal place they are on: 1000 has three zeroes to the left of the decimal, so insert three zeroes between the 5 and the decimal, or move the decimal place over three places to the right, for your answer of 5000 mL.

Example
How many kilograms are in 4.8 grams?

There is 1 gram for every 0.001 kilograms. Since there is one-thousandth of a kilogram for each gram, that means divide by 1000, or move the decimal to the left by 3 places – 1 place for each 0. So, the result would be 0.0048 kg.

For quick conversions, move the decimal place the set number of spaces left or right to match the column/slot, as depicted below.

To convert from one prefix to another to the left or right of the base unit (follow the arrow to the left or right), move the decimal place the number of columns/slots as counted.

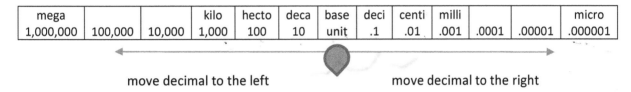

mega			kilo	hecto	deca	base	deci	centi	milli			micro
1,000,000	100,000	10,000	1,000	100	10	unit	.1	.01	.001	.0001	.00001	.000001

move decimal to the left   move decimal to the right

Example
How many centiliters are in 4.7 kiloliters?

To convert a number with a unit prefixed as kilo into a unit prefixed as centi, move across five columns to the right, meaning move the decimal place five places to the right.

$$4.7 \text{ kL} = 470,000 \text{ cL}$$

Example
How many liters are in 30 microliters?

Start with the unit marked micro and count the columns moving to the left until you reach the base unit for liters. Be sure to count the blank columns, as they are important placeholders. There are six columns from micro to the base unit moving to the left, so move the decimal place six places to the left.

$$30 \text{ mL} = 0.000030 \text{ L}$$

Decimal Addition

Addition with decimals is done the same way as regular addition. All numbers could have decimals, but are often removed if the numbers to the right of the decimal are zeros. Line up numbers at the decimal place.

Example: Add 345.89 + 23.54

Line the numbers up at the decimal place and add.

```
  3 4 5 . 8 9
+   2 3 . 5 4
-------------
  3 6 9 . 4 3
```

Decimal Subtraction

Subtraction with decimals is done the same way as regular subtraction.

Example: Subtract 345.89 − 23.54

Line the numbers up at the decimal place and subtract.

```
  3 4 5 . 8 9
-   2 3 . 5 4
-------------
  3 2 2 . 3 5
```

Decimal Multiplication

The simplest way to handle multiplication with decimals is to calculate the multiplication problem pretending the decimals are not there, then count how many decimal places there are in the original problem. Use that total to place the decimal the same number of places over, counting from right to left.

Example: Multiply 42.33 × 3.3

Line the numbers up and multiply, pretending there are no decimals.

```
        4 2 3 3
  x         3 3
  -------------
      1 2 6 9 9
    1 2 6 9 9 0
  -------------
    1 3 9 6 8 9
```

Now look at the original problem and count how many decimal places were removed. Two decimal places were removed from 42.33 to get 4233, and one decimal place from 3.3 to get 33. Removed were $2 + 1 = 3$ decimal places. Place the decimal three places from the right of the number 139689. The answer is 139.689.

Another way to think of this is that when you move the decimal in the original numbers, it is like multiplying by 10. To put the decimals back, you need to divide the number by 10 the same amount of times you multiplied. It would still be three times for the above solution.

Example: Multiply 0.03 × 1.22

Line the numbers up and multiply, pretending there are no decimals. The zeroes in front of the 3 are unnecessary, so take them out for now.

$$
\begin{array}{r}
1\ 2\ 2 \\
\times \qquad 3 \\
\hline
3\ 6\ 6
\end{array}
$$

Look at the original problem and count how many decimals places were removed, or how many times each number was multiplied by 10. The 1.22 moved two places (or multiplied by 10 twice), as did 0.03. That is $2 + 2 = 4$ decimal places removed. Count that number, from right to left of the number 366, and place the decimal. The result is 0.0366.

Decimal Division

Division with decimals is simplest when you eliminate some of the decimal places. Since you divide the bottom number of a fraction into the top, or divide the denominator into the numerator, the bottom number dictates the movement of the decimals. The goal is to remove the decimals from the denominator and mirror that movement in the numerator. You do not need the numerator to be decimal free, however. Divide as you would normally.

Example
Divide 4.21/0.2 or 4.21 ÷ 0.2

Move the decimal over one place to the right in the denominator, making 0.2 simply 2. Move the decimal in the numerator, 4.21, over the same amount, so it is now 42.1.

$$
0.2\overline{)4.21}
$$

Becomes

$$
2\overline{)42.1}
$$

Divide.

$$
\begin{array}{r}
21.05 \\
2\overline{)42.10}
\end{array}
$$

The answer is 21.05 with the correct decimal placement. In decimal division, move the decimal the same amount for both numerator and denominator. There is no need to adjust anything after the problem is completed.

Fractions

A fraction is an equation that represents a part of a whole, but can also be used to present ratios or division problems. An example of a fraction is $\frac{x}{y}$. In this example, x is called the **numerator**, while y is the **denominator**. The numerator represents the number of parts, and the denominator is the total number of parts. They are separated by a line or slash, known as a **fraction bar**. In simple fractions, the numerator and denominator can be nearly any integer. However, the denominator of a fraction can never be zero, because dividing by zero is a function which is undefined.

Imagine that an apple pie has been baked for a holiday party, and the full pie has eight slices. After the party, there are five slices left. How could the amount of the pie that remains be expressed as a fraction? The numerator is 5 since there are 5 pieces left, and the denominator is 8 since there were eight total slices in the whole pie. Thus, expressed as a fraction, the leftover pie totals $\frac{5}{8}$ of the original amount.

Fractions come in three different varieties: proper fractions, improper fractions, and mixed numbers. **Proper fractions** have a numerator less than the denominator, such as $\frac{3}{8}$, but **improper fractions** have a numerator greater than the denominator, such as $\frac{15}{8}$. **Mixed numbers** combine a whole number with a proper fraction, such as $3\frac{1}{2}$. Any mixed number can be written as an improper fraction by multiplying the integer by the denominator, adding the product to the value of the numerator, and dividing the sum by the original denominator. For example, $3\frac{1}{2} = \frac{3 \times 2 + 1}{2} = \frac{7}{2}$. Whole numbers can also be converted into fractions by placing the whole number as the numerator and making the denominator 1. For example, $3 = \frac{3}{1}$.

One of the most fundamental concepts of fractions is their ability to be manipulated by multiplication or division. This is possible since $\frac{n}{n} = 1$ for any non-zero integer. As a result, multiplying or dividing by $\frac{n}{n}$ will not alter the original fraction since any number multiplied or divided by 1 doesn't change the value of that number. Fractions of the same value are known as equivalent fractions. For example, $\frac{2}{4}, \frac{4}{8}, \frac{50}{100}$, and $\frac{75}{150}$ are equivalent, as they all equal $\frac{1}{2}$.

Although many equivalent fractions exist, they are easier to compare and interpret when reduced or simplified. The numerator and denominator of a simple fraction will have no factors in common other than 1. When reducing or simplifying fractions, divide the numerator and denominator by the **greatest common factor**. A simple strategy is to divide the numerator and denominator by low numbers, like 2, 3, or 5 until arriving at a simple fraction, but the same thing could be achieved by determining the greatest common factor for both the numerator and denominator and dividing each by it. Using the first method is preferable when both the numerator and denominator are even, end in 5, or are obviously a multiple of another number. However, if no numbers seem to work, it will be necessary to factor the numerator and denominator to find the GCF. Let's look at examples:

1) Simplify the fraction $\frac{6}{8}$:

Dividing the numerator and denominator by 2 results in $\frac{3}{4}$, which is a simple fraction.

2) Simplify the fraction $\frac{12}{36}$:

Dividing the numerator and denominator by 2 leaves $\frac{6}{18}$. This isn't a simple fraction, as both the numerator and denominator have factors in common. Diving each by 3 results in $\frac{2}{6}$, but this can be further simplified by dividing by 2 to get $\frac{1}{3}$. This is the simplest fraction, as the numerator is 1. In cases like this, multiple division operations can be avoided by determining the greatest common factor between the numerator and denominator.

3) Simplify the fraction $\frac{18}{54}$ by dividing by the greatest common factor:

First, determine the factors for the numerator and denominator. The factors of 18 are 1, 2, 3, 6, 9, and 18. The factors of 54 are 1, 2, 3, 6, 9, 18, 27, and 54. Thus, the greatest common factor is 18. Dividing $\frac{18}{54}$ by 18 leaves $\frac{1}{3}$, which is the simplest fraction. This method takes slightly more work, but it definitively arrives at the simplest fraction.

Operations with Fractions

Of the four basic operations that can be performed on fractions, the one which involves the least amount of work is multiplication. To multiply two fractions, simply multiply the numerators, multiply the denominators, and place the products as a fraction. Whole numbers and mixed numbers can also be expressed as a fraction, as described above, to multiply with a fraction. Let's work through a couple of examples.

1) $\frac{2}{5} \times \frac{3}{4} = \frac{6}{20} = \frac{3}{10}$

2) $\frac{4}{9} \times \frac{7}{11} = \frac{28}{99}$

Dividing fractions is similar to multiplication with one key difference. To divide fractions, flip the numerator and denominator of the second fraction, and then proceed as if it were a multiplication problem:

1) $\frac{7}{8} \div \frac{4}{5} = \frac{7}{8} \times \frac{5}{4} = \frac{35}{32}$

2) $\frac{5}{9} \div \frac{1}{3} = \frac{5}{9} \times \frac{3}{1} = \frac{15}{9} = \frac{5}{3}$

Addition and subtraction require more steps than multiplication and division, as these operations require the fractions to have the same denominator, also called a **common denominator**. It is always possible to find a common denominator by multiplying the denominators. However, when the denominators are large numbers, this method is unwieldy, especially if the answer must be provided in its simplest form. Thus, it's beneficial to find the **least common denominator** of the fractions—the least common denominator is incidentally also the least common multiple.

Once equivalent fractions have been found with common denominators, simply add or subtract the numerators to arrive at the answer:

1) $\frac{1}{2} + \frac{3}{4} = \frac{2}{4} + \frac{3}{4} = \frac{5}{4}$

2) $\frac{3}{12} + \frac{11}{20} = \frac{15}{60} + \frac{33}{60} = \frac{48}{60} = \frac{4}{5}$

3) $\frac{7}{9} - \frac{4}{15} = \frac{35}{45} - \frac{12}{45} = \frac{23}{45}$

4) $\frac{5}{6} - \frac{7}{18} = \frac{15}{18} - \frac{7}{18} = \frac{8}{18} = \frac{4}{9}$

Changing Fractions to Decimals

To change a fraction into a decimal, divide the denominator into the numerator until there are no remainders. There may be repeating decimals, so rounding is often acceptable. A straight line above the repeating portion denotes that the decimal repeats.

<u>Example</u>
Express 4/5 as a decimal.

Set up the division problem.

$$5\overline{)4}$$

5 does not go into 4, so place the decimal and add a zero.

$$5\overline{)4.0}$$

5 goes into 40 eight times. There is no remainder.

$$\begin{array}{r} 0.8 \\ 5\overline{)4.0} \\ -\ 4.0 \\ \hline 0 \end{array}$$

The solution is 0.8.

<u>Example</u>
Express 33 1/3 as a decimal.

Since the whole portion of the number is known, set it aside to calculate the decimal from the fraction portion.

Set up the division problem.

$$3\overline{)1}$$

3 does not go into 1, so place the decimal and add zeros. 3 goes into 10 three times.

$$\begin{array}{r} 0.3 \\ 3\overline{)1.0} \end{array}$$

This will repeat with a remainder of 1.

$$
\begin{array}{r}
0.333 \\
3\overline{)1.000} \\
-9 \\
\hline
10 \\
-9 \\
\hline
10
\end{array}
$$

So, we will place a line over the 3 to denote the repetition. The solution is written $33.\overline{3}$.

Changing Decimals to Fractions

To change decimals to fractions, place the decimal portion of the number, the numerator, over the respective place value, the denominator, then reduce, if possible.

<u>Example</u>
Express 0.25 as a fraction.

This is read as twenty-five hundredths, so put 25 over 100. Then reduce to find the solution.

$$
\frac{25}{100} = \frac{1}{4}
$$

<u>Example</u>
Express 0.455 as a fraction

This is read as four hundred fifty-five thousandths, so put 455 over 1000. Then reduce to find the solution.

$$
\frac{455}{1000} = \frac{91}{200}
$$

There are two types of problems that commonly involve percentages. The first is to calculate some percentage of a given quantity, where you convert the percentage to a decimal, and multiply the quantity by that decimal. Secondly, you are given a quantity and told it is a fixed percent of an unknown quantity. In this case, convert to a decimal, then divide the given quantity by that decimal.

<u>Example</u>
What is 30% of 760?

Convert the percent into a useable number. "Of" means to multiply.

$$
30\% = 0.30
$$

Set up the problem based on the givens, and solve.

$$
0.30 \times 760 = 228
$$

<u>Example</u>
8.4 is 20% of what number?

Convert the percent into a useable number.

$$20\% = 0.20$$

The given number is a percent of the answer needed, so divide the given number by this decimal rather than multiplying it.

$$\frac{8.4}{0.20} = 42$$

Ratios and Proportions

<u>Ratios</u>
Ratios are used to show the relationship between two quantities. The ratio of oranges to apples in the grocery store may be 3 to 2. That means that for every 3 oranges, there are 2 apples. This comparison can be expanded to represent the actual number of oranges and apples. Another example may be the number of boys to girls in a math class. If the ratio of boys to girls is given as 2 to 5, that means there are 2 boys to every 5 girls in the class. Ratios can also be compared if the units in each ratio are the same. The ratio of boys to girls in the math class can be compared to the ratio of boys to girls in a science class by stating which ratio is higher and which is lower.

Rates are used to compare two quantities with different units. *Unit rates* are the simplest form of rate. With **unit rates**, the denominator in the comparison of two units is one. For example, if someone can type at a rate of 1000 words in 5 minutes, then his or her unit rate for typing is $\frac{1000}{5} = 200$ words in one minute or 200 words per minute. Any rate can be converted into a unit rate by dividing to make the denominator one. 1000 words in 5 minutes has been converted into the unit rate of 200 words per minute.

Ratios and rates can be used together to convert rates into different units. For example, if someone is driving 50 kilometers per hour, that rate can be converted into miles per hour by using a ratio known as the **conversion factor.** Since the given value contains kilometers and the final answer needs to be in miles, the ratio relating miles to kilometers needs to be used. There are 0.62 miles in 1 kilometer. This, written as a ratio and in fraction form, is $\frac{0.62 \, miles}{1 \, km}$. To convert 50km/hour into miles per hour, the following conversion needs to be set up:

$$\frac{50 \, km}{hour} * \frac{0.62 \, miles}{1 \, km} = 31 \, miles \, per \, hour$$

The ratio between two similar geometric figures is called the **scale factor.** For example, a problem may depict two similar triangles, A and B. The scale factor from the smaller triangle A to the larger triangle B is given as 2 because the length of the corresponding side of the larger triangle, 16, is twice the corresponding side on the smaller triangle, 8. This scale factor can also be used to find the value of a missing side, x, in triangle A. Since the scale factor from the smaller triangle (A) to larger one (B) is 2, the larger corresponding side in triangle B (given as 25), can be divided by 2 to find the missing side in A ($x = 12.5$). The scale factor can also be represented in the equation $2A = B$ because two times the lengths of A gives the corresponding lengths of B. This is the idea behind similar triangles.

Proportions

Much like a scale factor can be written using an equation like $2A = B$, a **relationship** is represented by the equation $Y = kX$. X and Y are proportional because as values of X increase, the values of Y also increase. A relationship that is inversely proportional can be represented by the equation $Y = \frac{k}{x}$, where the value of Y decreases as the value of x increases and vice versa.

Proportional reasoning can be used to solve problems involving ratios, percentages, and averages. Ratios can be used in setting up proportions and solving them to find unknowns. For example, if a student completes an average of 10 pages of math homework in 3 nights, how long would it take the student to complete 22 pages? Both ratios can be written as fractions. The second ratio would contain the unknown.

The following proportion represents this problem, where x is the unknown number of nights:

$$\frac{10 \; pages}{3 \; nights} = \frac{22 \; pages}{x \; nights}$$

Solving this proportion entails cross-multiplying (multiplying both sets of numbers that are diagonally across and setting them equal to each other) and results in the following equation: $10x = 22 * 3$. Simplifying and solving for x results in the exact solution: $x = 6.6 \; nights$. The result would be rounded up to 7 because the homework would actually be completed on the 7th night.

The following problem uses ratios involving percentages:

If 20% of the class is girls and 30 students are in the class, how many girls are in the class?

To set up this problem, it is helpful to use the common proportion: $\frac{\%}{100} = \frac{is}{of}$. Within the proportion, % is the percentage of girls, 100 is the total percentage of the class, *is* is the number of girls, and *of* is the total number of students in the class. Most percentage problems can be written using this language. To solve this problem, the proportion should be set up as $\frac{20}{100} = \frac{x}{30}$, and then solved for x. Cross-multiplying results in the equation $20 * 30 = 100x$, which results in the solution $x = 6$. There are 6 girls in the class.

Problems involving volume, length, and other units can also be solved using ratios. For example, a problem may ask for the volume of a cone to be found that has a radius, $r = 7m$ and a height, $h = 16m$. Referring to the formulas provided on the test, the volume of a cone is given as: $V = \pi r^2 \frac{h}{3}$, where r is the radius, and h is the height. Plugging $r = 7$ and $h = 16$ into the formula, the following is obtained: $V = \pi (7^2) \frac{16}{3}$. Therefore, volume of the cone is found to be approximately 821m³. Sometimes, answers in different units are sought. If this problem wanted the answer in liters, 821m³ would need to be converted. Using the equivalence statement 1m³ = 1000L, the following ratio would be used to solve for liters: $821m^3 * \frac{1000L}{1m^3}$. Cubic meters in the numerator and denominator cancel each other out, and the answer is converted to 821,000 liters, or $8.21 * 10^5$ L.

Other conversions can also be made between different given and final units. If the temperature in a pool is 30°C, what is the temperature of the pool in degrees Fahrenheit? To convert these units, an equation is used relating Celsius to Fahrenheit. The following equation is used: $T_{°F} = 1.8T_{°C} + 32$. Plugging in the given temperature and solving the equation for T yields the result: $T_{°F} = 1.8(30) + 32 = 86°F$. Both units in the metric system and U.S. customary system are widely used.

Here are some more examples of how to solve for proportions:

1) $\frac{75\%}{90\%} = \frac{25\%}{x}$

To solve for x, the fractions must be cross multiplied: ($75\%x = 90\% \times 25\%$). To make things easier, let's convert the percentages to decimals: ($0.9 \times 0.25 = 0.225 = 0.75x$). To get rid of x's coefficient, each side must be divided by that same coefficient to get the answer $x = 0.3$. The question could ask for the answer as a percentage or fraction in lowest terms, which are 30% and $\frac{3}{10}$, respectively.

2) $\frac{x}{12} = \frac{30}{96}$

Cross-multiply: $96x = 30 \times 12$

Multiply: $96x = 360$

Divide: $x = 360 \div 96$

Answer: $x = 3.75$

3) $\frac{0.5}{3} = \frac{x}{6}$

Cross-multiply: $3x = 0.5 \times 6$

Multiply: $3x = 3$

Divide: $x = 3 \div 3$

Answer: $x = 1$

You may have noticed there's a faster way to arrive at the answer. If there is an obvious operation being performed on the proportion, the same operation can be used on the other side of the proportion to solve for x. For example, in the first practice problem, 75% became 25% when divided by 3, and upon doing the same to 90%, the correct answer of 30% would have been found with much less legwork. However, these questions aren't always so intuitive, so it's a good idea to work through the steps, even if the answer seems apparent from the outset.

Percentages

Think of percentages as fractions with a denominator of 100. In fact, **percentage** means "per hundred." Problems often require converting numbers from percentages, fractions, and decimals. The following explains how to work through those conversions.

Conversions

Decimals and Percentages: Since a percentage is based on "per hundred," decimals and percentages can be converted by multiplying or dividing by 100. Practically speaking, this always amounts to moving the decimal point two places to the right or left, depending on the conversion. To convert a percentage to a decimal, move the decimal point two places to the left and remove the % sign. To convert a decimal to a percentage, move the decimal point two places to the right and add a "%" sign. Here are some examples:

65% = 0.65
0.33 = 33%
0.215 = 21.5%
99.99% = 0.9999
500% = 5.00
7.55 = 755%

Fractions and Percentages: Remember that a percentage is a number per one hundred. So, a percentage can be converted to a fraction by making the number in the percentage the numerator and putting 100 as the denominator:

$$43\% = \frac{43}{100}$$

$$97\% = \frac{97}{100}$$

$$4.7\% = \frac{47}{1000}$$

Note in the last example, that the decimal can be removed by going from 100 to 1,000, because it's accomplished by multiplying the numerator and denominator by 10.

Note that the percent symbol (%) kind of looks like a 0, a 1, and another 0. So, think of a percentage like 54% as 54 over 100. Note that it's often good to simplify a fraction into the smallest possible numbers. So, 54/100 would then become 27/50:

$$\frac{54}{100} \div \frac{2}{2} = \frac{27}{50}$$

To convert a fraction to a percent, follow the same logic. If the fraction happens to have 100 in the denominator, you're in luck. Just take the numerator and add a percent symbol:

$$\frac{28}{100} = 28\%$$

Another option is to make the denominator equal to 100. Be sure to multiply the numerator by the same number as the denominator. For example:

$$\frac{3}{20} \times \frac{5}{5} = \frac{15}{100}$$

$$\frac{15}{100} = 15\%$$

If neither of those strategies work, divide the numerator by the denominator to get a decimal:

$$\frac{9}{12} = 0.75$$

Then convert the decimal to a percentage:

$$0.75 = 75\%$$

Percent Formula

The percent formula looks like this:

$$\frac{\textbf{part}}{\textbf{whole}} = \frac{\%}{\textbf{100}}$$

After numbers are plugged in, multiply the diagonal numbers and then divide by the remaining one. It works every time.

So, when a question asks what percent 5 is of 10. You plug the numbers in:

$$\frac{\textbf{5}}{\textbf{10}} = \frac{\%}{\textbf{100}}$$

Multiply the diagonal numbers:

$$5 \times 100 = 500$$

Divide by the remaining number:

$$\frac{500}{10} = 50\%$$

The percent formula can be applied in a number of different circumstances by plugging in the numbers appropriately.

Regular Time vs. Military Time

When telling time with a regular or 12-hour clock, start counting at 12 a.m., or midnight, increasing each hour by whole numbers: 1 a.m., 2 a.m., 3 a.m., and so on. Once the count reaches 12 again, it becomes 12 p.m., or noon, and the count goes from 1 p.m., 2 p.m., 3 p.m., and so on. This switching of a.m. to p.m. and back continues in a cycle. A colon is used to separate the hours from the minutes and the minutes from the seconds.

Military time uses a 24-hour clock. Military time also begins at midnight and continues on to 1, 2, 3, and so on. It does not use a.m. or p.m. Midnight is the 24th hour in the count. What regular time considers 1 a.m. is called 0100, pronounced "zero one hundred hours" or "oh one hundred hours," in military time. This continues for the entire count – 0200, 0300, 0400, etc. – until you reach what regular time calls 12 p.m. or 1200, pronounced "twelve hundred hours," and then continues the count to 1300, 1400, 1500, and so on. See the following for a comparison chart:

Regular	Military
12 a.m. Midnight	2400 Midnight/Twenty-four hundred hours
1 a.m. One o'clock	0100 Zero one hundred hours
2 a.m. Two o'clock	0200 Zero two hundred hours
3 a.m. Three o'clock	0300 Zero three hundred hours
4 a.m. Four o'clock	0400 Zero four hundred hours
5 a.m. Five o'clock	0500 Zero five hundred hours
6 a.m. Six o'clock	0600 Zero six hundred hours
7 a.m. Seven o'clock	0700 Zero seven hundred hours
8 a.m. Eight o'clock	0800 Zero eight hundred hours
9 a.m. Nine o'clock	0900 Zero nine hundred hours
10 a.m. Ten o'clock	1000 Ten hundred hours
11 a.m. Eleven o'clock	1100 Eleven hundred hours
12 p.m. Noon	1200 Noon/Twelve hundred hours
1 p.m. One o'clock	1300 Thirteen hundred hours
2 p.m. Two o'clock	1400 Fourteen hundred hours
3 p.m. Three o'clock	1500 Fifteen hundred hours
4 p.m. Four o'clock	1600 Sixteen hundred hours
5 p.m. Five o'clock	1700 Seventeen hundred hours
6 p.m. Six o'clock	1800 Eighteen hundred hours
7 p.m. Seven o'clock	1900 Nineteen hundred hours
8 p.m. Eight o'clock	2000 Twenty hundred hours
9 p.m. Nine o'clock	2100 Twenty-one hundred hours
10 p.m. Ten o'clock	2200 Twenty-two hundred hours
11 p.m. Eleven o'clock	2300 Twenty-three hundred hours

A trick for converting from military to regular time is if the time is twelve hundred hours or less, it is equivalent to the a.m. version in regular time. If the time is thirteen hundred hours or more, subtract twelve and add p.m. to convert it to regular time.

Example
You are to meet someone at fourteen hundred hours. Note that the military time is more than thirteen hundred, so subtract twelve from the time.

$$14 - 12 = 2 \, p.m.$$

Example
A person needs his medicine at twenty-three hundred hours. Note the military time is more than thirteen hundred, so subtract twelve from the time.

$$23 - 12 = 11 \, p.m.$$

Properties of Exponents

Exponents are used in mathematics to express a number or variable multiplied by itself a certain number of times. For example, x^3 means x is multiplied by itself three times. In this expression, x is called the **base**, and 3 is the exponent. Exponents can be used in more complex problems when they contain fractions and negative numbers.

Order of Operations

When solving equations with multiple operations, special rules apply. These rules are known as the **Order of Operations**. The order is as follows: Parentheses, Exponents, Multiplication and Division from left to right, and Addition and Subtraction from left to right. A popular mnemonic device to help remember the order is Please Excuse My Dear Aunt Sally (PEMDAS). Evaluate the following two problems to understand the Order of Operations:

1) $4 + (3 \times 2)^2 \div 4$

First, solve the operation within the parentheses: $4 + 6^2 \div 4$.
Second, solve the exponent: $4 + 36 \div 4$.
Third, solve the division operation: $4 + 9$.
Fourth, finish the operation with addition for the answer, 13.

2) $2 \times (6 + 3) \div (2 + 1)^2$

$2 \times 9 \div (3)^2$
$2 \times 9 \div 9$
$18 \div 9$
2

Algebra

Algebra is used to describe things in mathematics that have differing or changeable variables. It is easily applied to real-world situations, due to its versatility. Algebra often uses **variables**, which represent unknown quantities or values. Variables are usually represented by a letter, such as X or Y. These are helpful when attempting to solve story problems. In algebra, letters are sometimes used to symbolize fixed values. In this case, the letters are called constants.

Below are some basic tips for navigating algebra.

To ensure multiplication signs (x) and unknown variables (X) are not confused, parentheses are placed around an object in an equation to signify multiplication.

Example
6 x 5 is the same as writing 6 (5).

Eliminate the multiplication sign between numbers and variables. It is understood they are multiplied.

Example
3 (X) and 3 x X and 3X all signify the same thing.

The multiplication symbol is sometimes replaced by a dot.

Example
6 $\times$ 5 can be written as 6 $\cdot$ 5.

Solving Equations in One Variable
Solving equations in one variable is the process of isolating a variable on one side of the equation. For example, in $3x - 7 = 20$, the variable is $3x$, and it needs to be isolated. The numbers (also called **constants**) are -7 and 20. That means $3x$ needs to be on one side of the equals sign (either side is fine) and all the numbers need to be on the other side of the equals sign.

To accomplish this, the equation must be manipulated by performing opposite operations of what already exists. Remember that addition and subtraction are opposites and that multiplication and division are opposites. Any action taken to one side of the equation must be taken on the other side to maintain equality.

So, since the 7 is being subtracted, it can be moved to the right side of the equation by adding seven to both sides:

$$3x - 7 = 20$$

$$3x - 7 + 7 = 20 + 7$$

$$3x = 27$$

Now that the variable $3x$ is on one side and the constants (now combined into one constant) are on the other side, the 3 needs to be moved to the right side. 3 and x are being multiplied together, so 3 then needs to be divided from each side.

$$\frac{3x}{3} = \frac{27}{3}$$

$$x = 9$$

Now that x has been completely isolated, we know its value.

The solution is found to be $x = 9$. This solution can be checked for accuracy by plugging $x = 9$ in the original equation. After simplifying the equation, $20 = 20$ is found, which is a true statement:

$$3 \times 9 - 7 = 20$$

$$27 - 7 = 20$$

$$20 = 20$$

Equations that require solving for a variable (**algebraic equations**) come in many forms. Here are some more examples:

No number attached to the variable:

$$x + 8 = 20$$

$$x + 8 - 8 = 20 - 8$$

$$x = 12$$

Fraction in the variable:

$$\frac{1}{2}z + 24 = 36$$

$$\frac{1}{2}z + 24 - 24 = 36 - 24$$

$$\frac{1}{2}z = 12$$

Now we multiply the fraction by its inverse:

$$\frac{2}{1} \times \frac{1}{2}z = 12 \times \frac{2}{1}$$

$$z = 24$$

Multiple instances of x:

$$14x + x - 4 = 3x + 2$$

All instances of x can be combined.

$$15x - 4 = 3x + 2$$

$$15x - 4 + 4 = 3x + 2 + 4$$

$$15x = 3x + 6$$

$$15x - 3x = 3x + 6 - 3x$$

36

$$12x = 6$$

$$\frac{12x}{12} = \frac{6}{12}$$

$$x = \frac{1}{2}$$

<u>Evaluating Expressions</u>

Sometimes expressions have multiple variables. For example:

$$5x + y - z$$

If you know what the variable equals, you can plug those numbers in for the variables and then solve the problem.

$$x = 3$$
$$y = 2$$
$$z = -3$$

$5(3) + 2 - (-3)$	Plug in the numbers for the variables
$15 + 2 - (-3)$	Follow the order of operations and perform multiplication first.
$15 + 2 + 3$	Subtraction of a negative can be changed to addition of a positive.
20	Add the terms

Algebraic **expressions** are built out of monomials. A monomial is a variable raised to some power multiplied by a constant: ax^n, where a is any constant and n is a whole number. A constant is also a monomial.

A polynomial is a sum of monomials. An example of a polynomial includes $3x^4 + 2x^2 - x - 3$.

Roman Numerals

Another form of denoting number value is through **Roman numerals**, which utilizes a finite set of letters from the alphabet to represent numbers. This numbering system doesn't account for 0, decimal, or negative numbers.

See the table below:

Arabic Numeral	Roman Numeral
1	I
5	V
10	X
50	L
100	C
500	D
1,000	M

Arabic Numeral	Roman Numeral	Arabic Numeral	Roman Numeral
1	I	6	VI
2	II	7	VII
3	III	8	VIII
4	IV	9	IX
5	V	10	X

There are two important steps to accurately reading and writing in Roman numerals. First, any smaller number immediately preceding a larger number is deducted from the larger number. For example, XC equals 90, as 10 is less than 100, so it's subtracted, as in 100–10=90. Second, any smaller numbers after the largest one are added.

Here's an example: XLIII equals 43. In the first step, X is smaller than L, so its value is deducted from that of L, leaving 40. But the III to the right of the L is now added to the remaining 40, giving a result of 43.

Here are some more examples:

Example
XXX is what number?

Since it is the same number next to itself, add the values together.

$$10 + 10 + 10 = 30$$

Example
XL is what number?

Since X is smaller than L, and X is in front of L, it means L – X.

$$50 - 10 = 40$$

Example
ML is what number?

Since L is smaller than M, and L is after M, it means M + L.

$$1000 + 50 = 1050$$

Example
XXIX is what number?

There are two identical numbers next to each other (XX), so add them: 10 + 10 = 20. Next, there is a smaller number (I) in front of a larger number (X), so subtract those: 10 - 1 = 9. Finally, combine all portions to get the total 20 + 9 = 29.

<u>Example</u>
What is 1988 in Roman numerals?

Break down the number into columns; 1000 + 900 + 80 + 8 = 1988

1000 = M, 900 = CM, 80 = LXXX, 8 = VIII

Combine them from left to right to get the final solution: MCMLXXXVIII

Identifying Relative Sizes of Measurement Units

The United States customary system and the metric system each consist of distinct units to measure lengths and volume of liquids. The U.S. customary units for length, from smallest to largest, are: inch (in), foot (ft), yard (yd), and mile (mi). The metric units for length, from smallest to largest, are: millimeter (mm), centimeter (cm), decimeter (dm), meter (m), and kilometer (km). The relative size of each unit of length is shown below.

U.S. Customary	Metric	Conversion
12in = 1ft	10mm = 1cm	1in = 254cm
36in = 3ft = 1yd	10cm = 1dm(decimeter)	1m ≈ 3.28ft ≈ 1.09yd
5,280ft = 1,760yd = 1mi	100cm = 10dm = 1m	1mi ≈ 1.6km
	1000m = 1km	

The U.S. customary units for volume of liquids, from smallest to largest, are: fluid ounces (fl oz), cup (c), pint (pt), quart (qt), and gallon (gal). The metric units for volume of liquids, from smallest to largest, are: milliliter (mL), centiliter (cL), deciliter (dL), liter (L), and kiloliter (kL). The relative size of each unit of liquid volume is shown below.

U.S. Customary	Metric	Conversion
8fl oz = 1c	10mL = 1cL	1pt ≈ 0.473L
2c = 1pt	10cL = 1dL	1L ≈ 1.057qt
4c = 2pt = 1qt	1,000mL = 100cL = 10dL = 1L	1gal ≈ 3,785L
4qt = 1gal	1,000L = 1kL	

The U.S. customary system measures weight (how strongly Earth is pulling on an object) in the following units, from least to greatest: ounce (oz), pound (lb), and ton. The metric system measures mass (the quantity of matter within an object) in the following units, from least to greatest: milligram (mg), centigram (cg), gram (g), kilogram (kg), and metric ton (MT).

The relative sizes of each unit of weight and mass are shown below.

U.S. Measures of Weight	Metric Measures of Mass
16oz = 1lb	10mg = 1cg
2,000lb = 1 ton	100cg = 1g
	1,000g = 1kg
	1,000kg = 1MT

Please keep in mind that all word problems on the actual test may be hospital-related.

Practice Questions

1. Add 5,089 + 10,323
    a. 15,402
    b. 15,412
    c. 5,234
    d. 15,234

2. Add 103,678 + 487
    a. 103,191
    b. 103,550
    c. 104,265
    d. 104,165

3. Add 1.001 + 5.629
    a. 6.630
    b. 4.628
    c. 5.630
    d. 6.628

4. Add 143.77 + 5.2
    a. 138.57
    b. 148.97
    c. 138.97
    d. 148.57

5. Add and express in reduced form 5/12 + 4/9
    a. 9/17
    b. 1/3
    c. 31/36
    d. 3/5

6. Add and express in reduced form 14/33 + 10/11.
    a. 2/11
    b. 6/11
    c. 4/3
    d. 44/33

7. Subtract 9,576 – 891.
    a. 10,467
    b. 9,685
    c. 8,325
    d. 8,685

8. Subtract 112,076 – 1,243.
   a. 110,833
   b. 113,319
   c. 113,833
   d. 110,319

9. Subtract 50.888 – 13.091.
   a. 37.797
   b. 63.979
   c. 37.979
   d. 33,817

10. Subtract 701.1 – 52.33.
   a. 753.43
   b. 648.77
   c. 652.77
   d. 638.43

11. Subtract and express in reduced form 23/24 – 1/6.
   a. 22/18
   b. 11/9
   c. 19/24
   d. 4/5

12. Subtract and express in reduced form 43/45 – 11/15.
   a. 10/45
   b. 16/15
   c. 32/30
   d. 2/9

13. Multiply 578 × 15.
   a. 8,770
   b. 8,760
   c. 8,660
   d. 8,670

14. Multiply 13, 114 × 191.
   a. 2,504,774
   b. 250,477
   c. 150,474
   d. 2,514,774

15. Multiply 12.4 × 0.2.
   a. 12.6
   b. 2.48
   c. 12.48
   d. 2.6

16. Multiply 1,987 × 0.05.
    a. 9.935
    b. 99.35
    c. 993.5
    d. 999.35

17. Multiply and reduce 15/23 × 54/127.
    a. 810/2,921
    b. 81/292
    c. 69/150
    d. 810/2929

18. Multiply and reduce 54/55 × 5/9.
    a. 59/64
    b. 270/495
    c. 6/11
    d. 5/9

19. Divide, express with a remainder 1,202 ÷ 44.
    a. 27 2/7
    b. 2 7/22
    c. 7 2/7
    d. 27 7/22

20. Divide, express with a remainder 188 ÷ 16.
    a. 1 3/4
    b. 111 3/4
    c. 10 3/4
    d. 11 3/4

21. Divide 702 ÷ 2.6.
    a. 27
    b. 207
    c. 2.7
    d. 270

22. Divide 1,015 ÷ 1.4.
    a. 7,250
    b. 725
    c. 7.25
    d. 72.50

23. Divide and reduce 26/55 ÷ 26/11.
    a. 52/11
    b. 26/11
    c. 1/5
    d. 2/5

24. Divide and reduce 4/13 ÷ 27/169.
    a. 52/27
    b. 51/27
    c. 52/29
    d. 51/29

25. What number is MCDXXXII?
    a. 142
    b. 1642
    c. 1632
    d. 1432

26. What number is CCLI?
    a. 1111
    b. 1151
    c. 151
    d. 251

27. Express 111 in Roman numerals.
    a. CCI
    b. CXI
    c. DDI
    d. DXI

28. Express 515 in Roman numerals.
    a. CVI
    b. DCV
    c. DXV
    d. VDV

29. Convert 1300 hours into a 12-hour clock time.
    a. 1:00 p.m.
    b. 11:00 a.m.
    c. 1:00 a.m.
    d. 11:00 p.m.

30. Convert 0830 hours into a 12-hour clock time.
    a. 8:30 p.m.
    b. 8:30 a.m.
    c. 11:30 a.m.
    d. 11:30 p.m.

31. What time is 5:00 p.m. in military (24-hour clock) time?
    a. 1500 hours
    b. 1700 hours
    c. 0500 hours
    d. 0700 hours

32. What time is 11:00am in military (24-hour clock) time?
    a. 0100 hours
    b. 1100 hours
    c. 1200 hours
    d. 0200 hours

33. The hospital has a nurse to patient ratio of 1:25. If there are a maximum of 325 patients admitted at a time, how many nurses are there?
    a. 13 nurses
    b. 25 nurses
    c. 325 nurses
    d. 12 nurses

34. A hospital has a bed to room ratio of 2: 1. If there are 145 rooms, how many beds are there?
    a. 145 beds
    b. 2 beds
    c. 90 beds
    d. 290 beds

35. Solve for X: $\frac{2x}{5} - 1 = 59$.
    a. 60
    b. 145
    c. 150
    d. 115

36. A National Hockey League store in the state of Michigan advertises 50% off all items. Sales tax in Michigan is 6%. How much would a hat originally priced at $32.99 and a jersey originally priced at $64.99 cost during this sale? Round to the nearest penny.
    a. $97.98
    b. $103.86
    c. $51.93
    d. $48.99

37. Store brand coffee beans cost $1.23 per pound. A local coffee bean roaster charges $1.98 per 1 ½ pounds. How much more would 5 pounds from the local roaster cost than 5 pounds of the store brand?
    a. $0.55
    b. $1.55
    c. $1.45
    d. $0.45

38. Paint Inc. charges $2000 for painting the first 1,800 feet of trim on a house and $1.00 per foot for each foot after. How much would it cost to paint a house with 3125 feet of trim?
    a. $3125
    b. $2000
    c. $5125
    d. $3325

39. A bucket can hold 11.4 liters of water. A kiddie pool needs 35 gallons of water to be full. How many times will the bucket need to be filled to fill the kiddie pool?

    a. 12
    b. 35
    c. 11
    d. 45

40. In Jim's school, there are 3 girls for every 2 boys. There are 650 students in total. Using this information, how many students are girls?

    a. 260
    b. 130
    c. 65
    d. 390

41. Convert 0.351 to a percentage.

    a. 3.51%

    b. 35.1%

    c. $\frac{351}{100}$

    d. 0.00351%

42. Convert $\frac{2}{9}$ to a percentage.

    a. 22%
    b. 4.5%
    c. 450%
    d. 0.22%

43. Convert 57% to a decimal.

    a. 570
    b. 5.70
    c. 0.06
    d. 0.57

44. What is 3 out of 8 expressed as a percent?

    a. 37.5%
    b. 37%
    c. 26.7%
    d. 2.67%

45. What is 39% of 164?

    a. 63.96
    b. 23.78
    c. 6,396
    d. 2.38

46. 32 is 25% of what number?
    a. 64
    b. 128
    c. 12.65
    d. 8

47. Convert $\frac{5}{8}$ to a decimal to the nearest hundredth.
    a. 0.62
    b. 1.05
    c. 0.63
    d. 1.60

48. Change $3\frac{3}{5}$ to a decimal.
    a. 3.6
    b. 4.67
    c. 5.3
    d. 0.28

49. Change 0.56 to a fraction.
    a. 5.6/100
    b. 14/25
    c. 56/1000
    d. 56/10

50. Change 9.3 to a fraction.
    a. $9\frac{3}{7}$
    b. $\frac{903}{1000}$
    c. $\frac{9.03}{100}$
    d. $9\frac{3}{10}$

Answer Explanations

1. B: 15,412

Set up the problem and add each column, starting on the far right (ones). Add, carrying anything over 9 into the next column to the left. Solve from right to left.

2. D: 104,165

Set up the problem and add each column, starting on the far right (ones). Add, carrying anything over 9 into the next column to the left. Solve from right to left.

3. A: 6.630

Set up the problem, with the larger number on top and numbers lined up at the decimal. Add, carrying anything over 9 into the next column to the left. Solve from right to left.

4. B: 148.97

Set up the problem, with the larger number on top and numbers lined up at the decimal. Insert 0 in any blank spots to the right of the decimal as placeholders. Add, carrying anything over 9 into the next column to the left.

5. C: 31/36

Set up the problem and find a common denominator for both fractions.

$$\frac{5}{12} + \frac{4}{9}$$

Multiply each fraction across by 1 to convert to a common denominator.

$$\frac{5}{12} \times \frac{3}{3} + \frac{4}{9} \times \frac{4}{4}$$

Once over the same denominator, add across the top. The total is over the common denominator.

$$\frac{15 + 16}{36} = \frac{31}{36}$$

6. C: 4/3

Set up the problem and find a common denominator for both fractions.

$$\frac{14}{33} + \frac{10}{11}$$

Multiply each fraction across by 1 to convert to a common denominator

$$\frac{14}{33} \times \frac{1}{1} + \frac{10}{11} \times \frac{3}{3}$$

Once over the same denominator, add across the top. The total is over the common denominator.

$$\frac{14+30}{33}=\frac{44}{33}$$

Reduce by dividing both numerator and denominator by 11.

$$\frac{44 \div 11}{33 \div 11}=\frac{4}{3}$$

7. D: 8,685

Set up the problem, with the larger number on top. Begin subtracting with the far right column (ones). Borrow 10 from the column to the left, when necessary.

8. A: 110,833

Set up the problem, with the larger number on top. Begin subtracting with the far right column (ones). Borrow 10 from the column to the left, when necessary.

9. A: 37.797

Set up the problem, larger number on top and numbers lined up at the decimal. Begin subtracting with the far right column. Borrow 10 from the column to the left, when necessary.

10. B: 648.77

Set up the problem, with the larger number on top and numbers lined up at the decimal. Insert 0 in any blank spots to the right of the decimal as placeholders. Begin subtracting with the far right column. Borrow 10 from the column to the left, when necessary.

11. C: 19/24

Set up the problem and find a common denominator for both fractions.

$$\frac{23}{24}-\frac{1}{6}$$

Multiply each fraction across by 1 to convert to a common denominator.

$$\frac{23}{24} \times \frac{1}{1}-\frac{1}{6} \times \frac{4}{4}$$

Once over the same denominator, subtract across the top.

$$\frac{23-4}{24}=\frac{19}{24}$$

12. D: 2/9

Set up the problem and find a common denominator for both fractions.

$$\frac{43}{45}-\frac{11}{15}$$

Multiply each fraction across by 1 to convert to a common denominator.

$$\frac{43}{45} \times \frac{1}{1} - \frac{11}{15} \times \frac{3}{3}$$

Once over the same denominator, subtract across the top.

$$\frac{43 - 33}{45} = \frac{10}{45}$$

Reduce.

$$\frac{10 \div 5}{45 \div 5} = \frac{2}{9}$$

13. D: 8670

Line up the numbers (the number with the most digits on top) to multiply. Begin with the left column on top and the left column on bottom (8 × 5).

Move one column left on top and multiply by the far right column on the bottom. Remember to add the carry over after you multiply.

Starting on the far right column, on top, repeat this pattern for the next number left on the bottom. Write the answers below the first line of answers. Remember to begin with a zero placeholder.

Continue the pattern.

Add the answer rows together, making sure they are still lined up correctly.

14. A: 2,504,774

Line up the numbers (the number with the most digits on top) to multiply. Begin with the right column on top and the right column on bottom.

Move one column left on top and multiply by the far right column on the bottom. Remember to add the carry over after you multiply. Continue that pattern for each of the numbers on the top row.

Starting on the far right column on top repeat this pattern for the next number left on the bottom. Write the answers below the first line of answers; remember to begin with a zero placeholder. Continue for each number in the top row.

Starting on the far right column on top, repeat this pattern for the next number left on the bottom. Write the answers below the first line of answers. Remember to begin with zero placeholders.

Once completed, ensure the answer rows are lined up correctly, then add.

15. B: 2.48

Set up the problem, with the larger number on top. Multiply as if there are no decimal places. Add the answer rows together. Count the number of decimal places that were in the original numbers (1 + 1 = 2).

Place the decimal 2 places the right for the final solution.

16. B: 99.35

Set up the problem, with the larger number on top. Multiply as if there are no decimal places. Add the answer rows together. Count the number of decimal places that were in the original numbers (2).

Place the decimal in that many spots from the right for the final solution.

17. A: 810/2921

Line up the fractions.

$$\frac{15}{23} \times \frac{54}{127}$$

Multiply across the top and across the bottom.

$$\frac{15 \times 54}{23 \times 127} = \frac{810}{2921}$$

18. C: 6/11

Line up the fractions.

$$\frac{54}{55} \times \frac{5}{9}$$

Reduce fractions through cross-canceling.

$$\frac{6}{11} \times \frac{1}{1}$$

Multiply across the top and across the bottom.

$$\frac{6 \times 1}{11 \times 1} = \frac{6}{11}$$

19. D: 27 7/22

Set up the division problem.

$$44\overline{)1202}$$

44 does not go into 1 or 12 but will go into 120 so start there.

$$
\begin{array}{r}
27 \\
44\overline{)1202} \\
-88 \\
\hline
322 \\
-308 \\
\hline
14
\end{array}
$$

The answer is 27 14/44.

Reduce the fraction for the final answer.

27 7/22

20. D: 11 3/4

Set up the division problem.

$$16\overline{)188}$$

16 does not go into 1 but does go into 18 so start there.

$$
\begin{array}{r}
11 \\
16\overline{)188} \\
-\ 16 \\
\hline
28 \\
-\ 16 \\
\hline
12
\end{array}
$$

The result is 11 12/16

Reduce the fraction for the final answer.

11 3/4

21. D: 270

Set up the division problem.

$$2.6\overline{)702}$$

Move the decimal over one place to the right in both numbers.

$$26\overline{)7020}$$

26 does not go into 7 but does go into 70 so start there.

$$
\begin{array}{r}
270 \\
26\overline{)7020} \\
-\ 52 \\
\hline
182 \\
-\ 182 \\
\hline
0
\end{array}
$$

The result is 270

22. B: 725

Set up the division problem.

$$1.4\overline{)1015}$$

Move the decimal over one place to the right in both numbers.

$$14\overline{)10150}$$

14 does not go into 1 or 10 but does go into 101 so start there.

$$
\begin{array}{r}
725 \\
14\overline{)10150} \\
-98 \\
\hline
35 \\
-28 \\
\hline
70 \\
-70 \\
\hline
0
\end{array}
$$

The result is 725.

23. C: 1/5

Set up the division problem.

$$\frac{26}{55} \div \frac{26}{11}$$

Flip the second fraction and multiply.

$$\frac{26}{55} \times \frac{11}{26}$$

Simplify and reduce with cross multiplication.

$$\frac{1}{5} \times \frac{1}{1}$$

Multiply across the top and across the bottom.

$$\frac{1 \times 1}{5 \times 1} = \frac{1}{5}$$

24. A: 52/27

Set up the division problem.

$$\frac{4}{13} \div \frac{27}{169}$$

Flip the second fraction and multiply.

$$\frac{4}{13} \times \frac{169}{27}$$

Simplify and reduce with cross multiplication.

$$\frac{4}{1} \times \frac{13}{27}$$

Multiply across the top and across the bottom to solve.

$$\frac{4 \times 13}{1 \times 27} = \frac{52}{27}$$

25. D: 1432

Break down the roman numerals into parts.

MCDXXXII

M is equal to 1000.

C is before D and is smaller than D, so it means D - C.

CD = 500 - 100 = 400

Add the following:

XXX = 10 + 10 + 10 = 30

II = 1 + 1 = 2

Add all parts.

1000 + 400 + 30 + 2 = 1432

26. D: 251

Break down the roman numerals into parts.

CCLI

Add the following.

CC = 100 + 100 = 200

L = 50

I = 1

Add all parts.

200 + 50 + 1 = 251

27. B: CXI

Break down the number into parts.

111 = 100 + 10 + 1

100 is represented by C or 100 = C

10 is represented by X or 10 = X

1 is represented by 1 or 1 = I

Combine the Roman numerals.

CXI

28. C: DXV

Break down the number into parts.

515 = 500 + 10 + 5

500 is represented by D or 500 = D

10 is represented by X or 10 = X

5 is represented by V or 5 = V

Combine the Roman numerals.

DXV

29. A: 1:00 p.m.

Since military time starts with 0100 at 1:00 a.m., add 12 to get to 1300 hours, or 1:00 p.m.

30. B: 8:30 a.m.

Anything before 1200 would be in the a.m. hours of a 12-hour clock, so 0830 hours is 8:30 a.m.

31. B: 1700 hours

To convert 5:00 p.m. into 24-hour time, add 12 to 5.

32. B: 1100 hours

Anything before noon converts into its a.m. value.

33. A: 13 nurses

Using the given information of 1 nurse to 25 patients and 325 patients, set up an equation to solve for number of nurses (N):

$$\frac{N}{325} = \frac{1}{25}$$

Multiply both sides by 325 to get N by itself on one side.

$$\frac{N}{1} = \frac{325}{25} = 13 \ nurses$$

34. D: 290 beds

Using the given information of 2 beds to 1 room and 145 rooms, set up an equation to solve for number of beds (B):

$$\frac{B}{145} = \frac{2}{1}$$

Multiply both sides by 145 to get B by itself on one side.

$$\frac{B}{1} = \frac{290}{1} = 290 \ beds$$

35. C: X = 150

Set up the initial equation.

$$\frac{2X}{5} - 1 = 59$$

Add 1 to both sides.

$$\frac{2X}{5} - 1 + 1 = 59 + 1$$

Multiply both sides by 5/2.

$$\frac{2X}{5} \times \frac{5}{2} = 60 \times \frac{5}{2} = 150$$

$$X = 150$$

36. C: $51.93

List the givens.

$$Tax = 6.0\% = 0.06$$

$$Sale = 50\% = 0.5$$

$$Hat = \$32.99$$

$$Jersey = \$64.99$$

Calculate the sales prices.

$$Hat\ Sale\ =\ 0.5\ (32.99)\ =\ 16.495$$

$$Jersey\ Sale\ =\ 0.5\ (64.99)\ =\ 32.495$$

Total the sales prices.

$$Hat\ sale\ +\ jersey\ sale\ =\ 16.495\ +\ 32.495\ =\ 48.99$$

Calculate the tax and add it to the total sales prices.

$$Total\ after\ tax\ =\ 48.99\ +\ (48.99\ x\ 0.06)\ =\ \$51.93$$

37. D: $0.45

List the givens.

$$Store\ coffee\ =\ \$1.23/lbs$$

$$Local\ roaster\ coffee\ =\ \$1.98/1.5\ lbs$$

Calculate the cost for 5 lbs of store brand.

$$\frac{\$1.23}{1\ lbs}\ \times 5\ lbs\ =\ \$6.15$$

Calculate the cost for 5 lbs of the local roaster.

$$\frac{\$1.98}{1.5\ lbs}\ \times 5\ lbs\ =\ \$6.60$$

Subtract to find the difference in price for 5 lbs.

$$\begin{array}{r} \$6.60 \\ -\$6.15 \\ \hline \$0.45 \end{array}$$

38. D: $3,325

List the givens.

$$1,800\ ft.=\ \$2,000$$

$$Cost\ after\ 1,800\ ft.=\ \$1.00/ft.$$

Find how many feet left after the first 1,800 ft.

$$\begin{array}{r} 3,125\ ft. \\ -\quad 1,800\ ft. \\ \hline 1,325\ ft. \end{array}$$

Calculate the cost for the feet over 1,800 ft.

$$1{,}325\ ft. \times \frac{\$1.00}{1\ ft} = \$1{,}325$$

Total for entire cost.

$$\$2{,}000 + \$1{,}325 = \$3{,}325$$

39. A: 12

Calculate how many gallons the bucket holds.

$$11.4\ L \ \times \ \frac{1\ gal}{3.8\ L} = 3\ gal$$

Now how many buckets to fill the pool which needs 35 gallons.

$$35/3 = 11.67$$

Since the amount is more than 11 but less than 12, we must fill the bucket 12 times.

40. D: Three girls for every two boys can be expressed as a ratio: 3:2. This can be visualized as splitting the school into 5 groups: 3 girl groups and 2 boy groups. The number of students which are in each group can be found by dividing the total number of students by 5:

650 divided by 5 equals 1 part, or 130 students per group

To find the total number of girls, multiply the number of students per group (130) by how the number of girl groups in the school (3). This equals 390, answer D.

41. B: 35.1%

To convert from a decimal to a percentage, the decimal needs to be moved two places to right. In this case, that makes 0.351 become 35.1%.

42. A: 22%

Converting from a fraction to a percentage generally involves two steps. First, the fraction needs to be converted to a decimal.

Divide 2 by 9 which results in $0.\overline{22}$. The top line indicates that the decimal actually goes on forever with an endless amount of 2's.

Second, the decimal needs to be moved two places to the right:

$$22\%$$

43. D: 0.57

To convert from a percentage to a decimal, or vice versa, you always need to move the decimal two places. A percentage like 57% has an invisible decimal after the 7, like this:

$$57.\%$$

That decimal then needs to be moved two places to the left to get:

$$0.57$$

44. A: 37.5%

Solve this by setting up the percent formula:

$$\frac{3}{8} = \frac{\%}{100}$$

Multiply 3 by 100 to get 300 . Then divide 300 by 8:

$$300 \div 8 = 37.5\%$$

Note that with the percent formula, 37.5 is automatically a percentage and does not need to have any further conversions.

45. A: 63.96%

This question involves the percent formula. Since, we're beginning with a percent, also known as a number over 100, we'll put 39 on the right side of the equation:

$$\frac{x}{164} = \frac{39}{100}$$

Now, multiple 164 and 39 to get 6,396, which then needs to be divided by 100.

$$6,396 \div 100 = 63.96$$

46. B: 128

This question involves the percent formula.

$$\frac{32}{x} = \frac{25}{100}$$

We multiply the diagonal numbers, 32 and 100, to get 3,200. Dividing by the remaining number, 25, gives us 128.

The percent formula does not have to be used for a question like this. Since 25% is ¼ of 100, you know that 32 needs to be multiplied by 4, which yields 128.

47. C: 0.63

Divide 5 by 8, which results in 0.625. This rounds up to 0.63.

48. A: 3.6

Divide 3 by 5 to get 0.6 and add that to the whole number 3, to get 3.6. An alternative is to incorporate the whole number 3 earlier on by creating an improper fraction: 18/5. Then dividing 18 by 5 to get 3.6.

49. B: 14/25

Since 0.56 goes to the hundredths place, it can be placed over 100:

$$\frac{56}{100}$$

Essentially, the way we got there is by multiplying the numerator and denominator by 100:

$$\frac{0.56}{1} \times \frac{100}{100} = \frac{56}{100}$$

Then, the fraction can be simplified down to 14/25:

$$\frac{56}{100} \div \frac{4}{4} = \frac{14}{25}$$

50. D: $9\frac{3}{10}$

To convert a decimal to a fraction, remember that any number to the left of the decimal point will be a whole number. Then, since 0.3 goes to the tenths place, it can be placed over 10.

Reading Comprehension

Identifying the Main Idea

Topics and main ideas are critical parts of any writing. The **topic** is the subject matter of the piece, and it is a broader, more general term. The **main idea** is what the writer wants to say about that topic. The topic can be expressed in a word or two, but the main idea should be a complete thought.

The topic and main idea are usually easy to recognize in nonfiction writing. An author will likely identify the topic immediately in the first sentence of a passage or essay. The main idea is also typically presented in the introductory paragraph of an essay. In a single passage, the main idea may be identified in the first or the last sentence, but will likely be directly stated and easily recognized by the reader. Because it is not always stated immediately in a passage, it's important to carefully read the entire passage to identify the main idea.

Also remember that when most authors write, they want to make a point or send a message. This point or message of a text is known as the theme. Authors may state themes explicitly, like in *Aesop's Fables*. More often, especially in modern literature, readers must infer the theme based on text details. Usually after carefully reading and analyzing an entire text, the theme emerges. Typically, the longer the piece, the more themes you will encounter, though often one theme dominates the rest, as evidenced by the author's purposeful revisiting of it throughout the passage.

The main idea should not be confused with the thesis statement. A thesis statement is a clear statement of the writer's specific stance, and can often be found in the introduction of a nonfiction piece. The main idea is more of an overview of the entire piece, while the thesis is a specific sentence found in that piece.

In order to illustrate the main idea, a writer will use **supporting details** in a passage. These details can provide evidence or examples to help make a point. Supporting details are most commonly found in nonfiction pieces that seek to inform or persuade the reader.

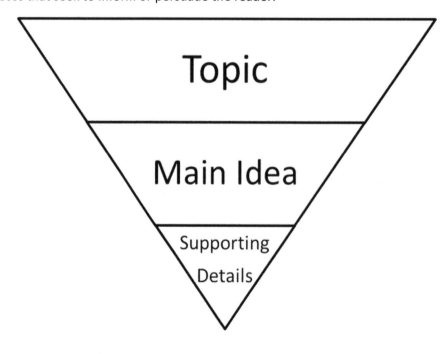

As a reader, you will want to carefully examine the author's supporting details to be sure they are credible. Consider whether they provide evidence of the author's point and whether they directly support the main idea. You might find that an author has used a shocking statistic to grab your attention, but that the statistic doesn't really support the main idea, so it isn't being effectively used in the piece.

Identifying Supporting Details

Supporting details help readers better develop and understand the main idea. Supporting details answer questions like *who, what, where, when, why,* and *how.* Different types of supporting details include examples, facts and statistics, anecdotes, and sensory details.

Persuasive and informative texts often use supporting details. In persuasive texts, authors attempt to make readers agree with their points of view, and supporting details are often used as "selling points." If authors make a statement, they need to support the statement with evidence in order to adequately persuade readers. Informative texts use supporting details such as examples and facts to inform readers. Review the previous "Cheetahs" passage to find examples of supporting details.

Cheetahs

Cheetahs are one of the fastest mammals on the land, reaching up to 70 miles an hour over short distances. Even though cheetahs can run as fast as 70 miles an hour, they usually only have to run half that speed to catch up with their choice of prey. Cheetahs cannot maintain a fast pace over long periods of time because their bodies will overheat. After a chase, cheetahs need to rest for approximately 30 minutes prior to eating or returning to any other activity.

In the example, supporting details include:

- Cheetahs reach up to 70 miles per hour over short distances.
- They usually only have to run half that speed to catch up with their prey.
- Cheetahs will overheat if they exert a high speed over longer distances.
- Cheetahs need to rest for 30 minutes after a chase.

Look at the diagram below (applying the cheetah example) to help determine the hierarchy of topic, main idea, and supporting details.

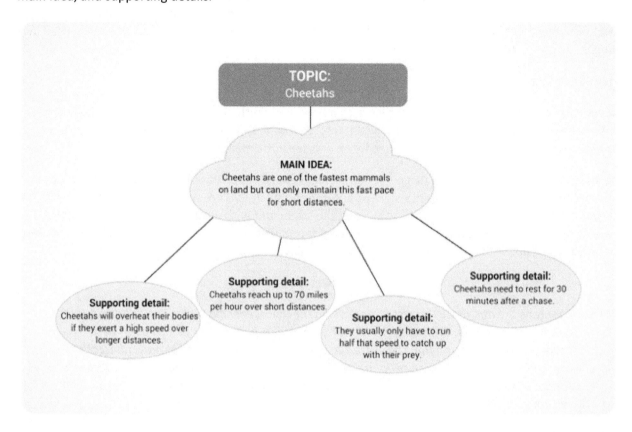

Finding the Meaning of Words and Phrases in Context

There will be many occasions in one's reading career in which an unknown word or a word with multiple meanings will pop up. There are ways of determining what these words or phrases mean that do not require the use of the dictionary, which is especially helpful during a test where one may not be available. Even outside of the exam, knowing how to derive an understanding of a word via **context clues** will be a critical skill in the real world. The context is the circumstances in which a story or a passage is happening, and can usually be found in the series of words directly before or directly after the word or phrase in question. The clues are the words that hint towards the meaning of the unknown word or phrase. The author may use synonyms or antonyms that you can use. **Synonyms** refer to words that have the same meaning as another word (e.g., instructor/teacher/educator, canine/dog, feline/cat, herbivore/vegetarian). **Antonyms** refer to words that have the opposite meaning as another word (e.g., true/false, up/down, in/out, right/wrong).

There may be questions that ask about the meaning of a particular word or phrase within a passage. There are a couple ways to approach these kinds of questions:

- Define the word or phrase in a way that is easy to comprehend (using context clues).
- Try out each answer choice in place of the word.

To demonstrate, here's an example from *Alice in Wonderland*:

> Alice was beginning to get very tired of sitting by her sister on the bank, and of having nothing to do: once or twice she <u>peeped</u> into the book her sister was reading, but it had no pictures or conversations in it, "and what is the use of a book," thought Alice, "without pictures or conversations?"

Q: As it is used in the selection, the word <u>peeped</u> means:

Using the first technique, before looking at the answers, define the word "peeped" using context clues and then find the matching answer. Then, analyze the entire passage in order to determine the meaning, not just the surrounding words.

To begin, imagine a blank where the word should be and put a synonym or definition there: "once or twice she ___ into the book her sister was reading." The context clue here is the book. It may be tempting to put "read" where the blank is, but notice the preposition word, "into." One does not read *into* a book, one simply reads a book, and since reading a book requires that it is seen with a pair of eyes, then "look" would make the most sense to put into the blank: "once or twice she <u>looked </u>into the book her sister was reading."

Once an easy-to-understand word or synonym has been supplanted, check to make sure it makes sense with the rest of the passage. What happened after she looked into the book? She thought to herself how a book without pictures or conversations is useless. This situation in its entirety makes sense.

Now check the answer choices for a match:
   a. To make a high-pitched cry
   b. To smack
   c. To look curiously
   d. To pout

Since the word was already defined, answer choice (c) is the best option.

Using the second technique, replace the figurative blank with each of the answer choices and determine which one is the most appropriate. Remember to look further into the passage to clarify that they work, because they could still make sense out of context.

Once or twice she <u>made a high pitched cry</u> into the book her sister was reading.

Once or twice she <u>smacked </u>the book her sister was reading.

Once or twice she <u>looked curiously</u> into the book her sister was reading.

Once or twice she <u>pouted</u> into the book her sister was reading.

For Choice *A*, it does not make much sense in any context for a person to yell into a book, unless maybe something terrible has happened in the story. Given that afterward Alice thinks to herself how useless a book without pictures is, this option does not make sense within context.

For Choice *B*, smacking a book someone is reading may make sense if the rest of the passage indicates there a reason for doing so. If Alice was angry or her sister had shoved it in her face, then maybe smacking the book would make sense within context. However, since whatever she does with the book causes her to think, "what is the use of a book without pictures or conversations?" then answer Choice *B* is not an appropriate answer.

Answer Choice *C* fits well within context, given her subsequent thoughts on the matter.

Answer Choice *D* does not make sense in context or grammatically, as people do not "pout into" things.

This is a simple example to illustrate the techniques outlined above. There may, however, be a question in which all of the definitions are correct and also make sense out of context, in which the appropriate context clues will really need to be honed in on in order to determine the correct answer. For example, here is another passage from *Alice in Wonderland*:

> ... but when the Rabbit actually took a watch out of its waistcoat pocket, and looked at it, and then hurried on, Alice <u>started</u> to her feet, for it flashed across her mind that she had never before seen a rabbit with either a waistcoat-pocket or a watch to take out of it, and burning with curiosity, she ran across the field after it, and was just in time to see it pop down a large rabbit-hole under the hedge.

Q: As it is used in the passage, the word <u>started</u> means:
   a. To turn on
   b. To begin
   c. To move quickly
   d. To be surprised

All of these words qualify as a definition of start, but using context clues, the correct answer can be identified using one of the two techniques above. It's easy to see that one does not turn on, begin, or be surprised to one's feet. The selection also states that she "ran across the field after it," indicating that she was in a hurry. Therefore, to move quickly would make the most sense in this context.

The same strategies can be applied to vocabulary that may be completely unfamiliar. In this case, focus on the words before or after the unknown word in order to determine its definition. Take this sentence, for example:

"Sam was such a <u>miser</u> that he forced Andrew to pay him twelve cents for the candy, even though he had a large inheritance and he knew his friend was poor."

Unlike with assertion questions, for vocabulary questions, it may be necessary to apply some critical thinking skills that may not be explicitly stated within the passage. Think about the implications of the passage, or what the text is trying to say. With this example, it is important to realize that it is considered unusually stingy for a person to demand so little money from someone instead of just letting their friend have the candy, especially if this person is already wealthy. Hence, a <u>miser</u> is a greedy or stingy individual.

Questions about complex vocabulary may not be explicitly asked, but this is a useful skill to know. If there is an unfamiliar word while reading a passage and its definition goes unknown, it is possible to miss out on a critical message that could inhibit the ability to appropriately answer the questions. Practicing this technique in daily life will sharpen this ability to derive meanings from context clues with ease.

Identifying a Writer's Purpose and Tone

<u>Purpose</u>

Writing can be classified under four passage types: narrative, expository, descriptive (sometimes called technical), and persuasive. Though these types are not mutually exclusive, one form tends to dominate the rest. By recognizing the *type* of passage you're reading, you gain insight into *how* you should read. If you're reading a narrative, you can assume the author intends to entertain, which means you may skim the text without losing meaning. A technical document might require a close read, because skimming the passage might cause the reader to miss salient details.

1. **Narrative writing**, at its core, is the art of storytelling. For a narrative to exist, certain elements must be present. It must have characters. While many characters are human, characters could be defined as anything that thinks, acts, and talks like a human. For example, many recent movies, such as *Lord of the Rings* and *The Chronicles of Narnia*, include animals, fantastical creatures, and even trees that behave like humans. It must have a plot or sequence of events. Typically, those events follow a standard plot diagram, but recent trends start *in medias res* or in the middle (near the climax). In this instance, foreshadowing and flashbacks often fill in plot details. Along with characters and a plot, there must also be conflict. Conflict is usually divided into two types: internal and external. Internal conflict indicates the character is in turmoil. Internal conflicts are presented through the character's thoughts. External conflicts are visible. Types of external conflict include a person versus nature, another person, and society.

2. **Expository writing** is detached and to the point. Since expository writing is designed to instruct or inform, it usually involves directions and steps written in second person ("you" voice) and lacks any persuasive or narrative elements. Sequence words such as *first*, *second*, and *third*, or *in the first place*, *secondly*, and *lastly* are often given to add fluency and cohesion. Common examples of expository writing include instructor's lessons, cookbook recipes, and repair manuals.

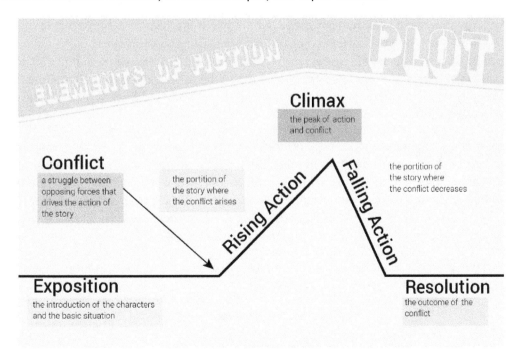

3. Due to its empirical nature, **technical writing** is filled with steps, charts, graphs, data, and statistics. The goal of technical writing is to advance understanding in a field through the scientific method.

Experts such as teachers, doctors, or mechanics use words unique to the profession in which they operate. These words, which often incorporate acronyms, are called *jargon*. Technical writing is a type of expository writing but is not meant to be understood by the general public. Instead, technical writers assume readers have received a formal education in a particular field of study and need no explanation as to what the jargon means. Imagine a doctor trying to understand a diagnostic reading for a car or a mechanic trying to interpret lab results. Only professionals with proper training will fully comprehend the text.

4. **Persuasive writing** is designed to change opinions and attitudes. The topic, stance, and arguments are found in the thesis, positioned near the end of the introduction. Later supporting paragraphs offer relevant quotations, paraphrases, and summaries from primary or secondary sources, which are then interpreted, analyzed, and evaluated. The goal of persuasive writers is not to stack quotes, but to develop original ideas by using sources as a starting point. Good persuasive writing makes powerful arguments with valid sources and thoughtful analysis. Poor persuasive writing is riddled with bias and logical fallacies. Sometimes, logical and illogical arguments are sandwiched together in the same piece. Therefore, readers should display skepticism when reading persuasive arguments.

Tone

Tone refers to the writer's attitude toward the subject matter. Tone is usually explained in terms of a work of fiction. For example, the tone conveys how the writer feels about the characters and the situations in which they're involved. Nonfiction writing is sometimes thought to have no tone at all; however, this is incorrect.

A lot of nonfiction writing has a neutral tone, which is an important one for the writer to use. A **neutral tone** demonstrates that the writer is presenting a topic impartially and letting the information speak for itself. On the other hand, nonfiction writing can be just as effective and appropriate if the tone isn't neutral. The following short passage provides an example of tone in nonfiction writing:

> Seat belts save more lives than any other automobile safety feature. Many studies show that airbags save lives as well; however, not all cars have airbags. For instance, some older cars don't. Furthermore, air bags aren't entirely reliable. For example, studies show that in 15% of accidents airbags don't deploy as designed, but, on the other hand, seat belt malfunctions are extremely rare. The number of highway fatalities has plummeted since laws requiring seat belt usage were enacted.

In this passage, the writer mostly chooses to retain a neutral tone when presenting information. If instead, the author chose to include his or her own personal experience of losing a friend or family member in a car accident, the tone would change dramatically. The tone would no longer be neutral and would show that the writer has a personal stake in the content, allowing him or her to interpret the information in a different way. When analyzing tone, the reader should consider what the writer is trying to achieve in the text and how they *create* the tone using style.

The following two poems and the essay concern the theme of death and are presented to demonstrate how to evaluate tone:

"Queen Mab," Percy Bysshe Shelley

How wonderful is Death,

Death, and his brother Sleep!

One, pale as yonder waning moon

With lips of lurid blue;

The other, rosy as the morn

When throned on ocean's wave

It blushes o'er the world;

Yet both so passing wonderful!

"After Great Pain, A Formal Feeling Comes," Emily Dickinson

After great pain, a formal feeling comes –

The Nerves sit ceremonious, like Tombs –

The stiff Heart questions 'was it He, that bore,'

And 'Yesterday, or Centuries before'?

The Feet, mechanical, go round –

A Wooden way

Of Ground, or Air, or Ought –

Regardless grown,

A Quartz contentment, like a stone –

This is the Hour of Lead –

Remembered, if outlived,

As Freezing persons, recollect the Snow –

First – Chill – then Stupor – then the letting go –

The Process of Dying

Death occurs in several stages. The first stage is the pre-active stage, which occurs a few days to weeks before death, in which the desire to eat and drink decreases, and the person may feel restless, irritable, and anxious. The second stage is the active stage, where the skin begins to cool, breathing becomes difficult as the lungs become congested (known as the "death rattle"), and the person loses control of their bodily fluids.

Once death occurs, there are also two stages. The first is clinical death, when the heart stops pumping blood and breathing ceases. This stage lasts approximately 4-6 minutes, and during this time, it is possible for a victim to be resuscitated via CPR or a defibrillator. After 6 minutes however, the oxygen stores within the brain begin to deplete, and the victim enters biological death. This is the point of no return, as the cells of the brain and vital organs begin to die, a process that is irreversible.

Readers should notice the differences in the word choices between the two poems. Percy Shelley's word choices—"wonderful," "rosy," "blushes," "ocean"—surrounding death indicates that he views death in a welcoming manner as his words carry positive charges. However, Dickinson's word choices—"pain," "wooden," "stone," "lead," "chill," "tombs"—carry negative connotations, which indicates an aversion to death. **Connotation** refers to the implied meaning of a word or phrase. Connotations are the ideas or feelings that words or phrase invoke other than their literal meaning. In contrast, the expository passage has no emotionally-charged words of any kind, and seems to view death simply as a process that happens, neither welcoming nor fearing it. The tone in this passage, therefore, is neutral.

Distinguishing between Fact and Opinion

It is important to distinguish between fact and opinion when reading a piece of writing. Readers should check the validity and accuracy of the facts that an author presents. When authors use opinion, they are sharing their own thoughts and feelings about the subject. You can recognize a piece that relies on opinion when the author uses words like *think, feel, believe,* or *in my opinion,* though these words won't always appear in an opinion piece, especially if it is formally written. An author's opinion may be backed up by facts, which gives it more credibility, but it should not be taken as fact. A critical reader should be suspect of an author's opinion, especially if it is only supported by other opinions.
Here are some examples of facts versus opinions:

Facts	Opinions
There are 9 innings in a game of baseball.	Baseball games run too long.
Eisenhower expanded Social Security.	This action was helpful for the country.
McDonalds has stores in 118 countries.	McDonalds has the best hamburgers.

As a critical reader, you must examine the facts that are used to support the author's argument. You can check the facts against other sources to be sure they are correct. You can also check the validity of the sources used to be sure they are credible, academic, and peer reviewed sources. Consider that when an author uses another person's opinion to support the argument, even if it is an expert's opinion, it is still only an opinion, and should not be taken as fact. A strong argument uses valid, measurable facts to support ideas. Even then, the reader may disagree with the argument, as it is rooted in the author's **assumptions**, which are the author's personal beliefs.

Making Logical Inferences

Critical readers should be able to make inferences. Making an **inference** requires the reader to read between the lines and look for what is *implied* rather than what is directly stated. That is, using information that *is* known from the text, the reader is able to make a logical assumption about information that is *not* directly stated but is probably true. Read the following passage:

"Hey, do you wanna meet my new puppy?" Jonathan asked.

"Oh, I'm sorry but please don't—" Jacinta began to protest, but before she could finish Jonathan had already opened the passenger side door of his car and a perfect white ball of fur came bouncing towards Jacinta.

"Isn't he the cutest?" beamed Jonathan.

"Yes—achoo!—he's pretty—aaaachooo!!—adora—aaa—aaaachoo!" Jacinta managed to say in between sneezes. "But if you don't mind, I—I—achoo!—need to go inside."

Which of the following can be inferred from Jacinta's reaction to the puppy?
a. she hates animals
b. she is allergic to dogs
c. she prefers cats to dogs
d. she is angry at Jonathan

An inference requires the reader to consider the information presented and then form their own idea about what is probably true. Based on the details in the passage, what is the best answer to the question? Important details to pay attention to include the tone of Jacinta's dialogue, which is overall polite and apologetic, as well as her reaction itself, which is a long string of sneezes. Answer Choices *A* and *D* both express strong emotions ("hates" and "angry") that are not evident in Jacinta's speech or actions. Answer Choice *C* mentions cats, but there is nothing in the passage to indicate Jacinta's feelings about cats. Answer Choice *B*, "she is allergic to dogs," is the most logical choice—based on the fact that she began sneezing as soon as a fluffy dog approached her, it makes sense to guess that Jacinta might be allergic to dogs. So even though Jacinta never directly states, "Sorry, I'm allergic to dogs!" using the clues in the passage, it is still reasonable to guess that this is true.

Making inferences is crucial for readers of literature, because literary texts often avoid presenting complete and direct information to readers about characters' thoughts or feelings, or they present this information in an unclear way, leaving it up to the reader to interpret clues given in the text. In order to make inferences while reading, readers should ask themselves:

- What details are being presented in the text?
- Is there any important information that seems to be missing?
- Based on the information that the author *does* include, what else is probably true?
- Is this inference reasonable based on what is already known?

Summarizing

A **summary** is a shortened version of the original text. It focuses on the main points of the original text and includes only the relevant details. Since summaries are generally significantly shorter than the text they are about, summaries need to get straight to the point. It's important that a summary retain the original meaning of the text. Generally, a summary should follow the flow of the passage by explaining the points in the same order as the originally passage; however, this is not a necessity.

Please keep in mind that passages found in the actual exam may be hospital-related.

Practice Questions

Questions 1-6 are based on the following passage:

When researchers and engineers undertake a large-scale scientific project, they may end up making discoveries and developing technologies that have far wider uses than originally intended. This is especially true in NASA, one of the most influential and innovative scientific organizations in America. NASA *spinoff technology* refers to innovations originally developed for NASA space projects that are now used in a wide range of different commercial fields. Many consumers are unaware that products they are buying are based on NASA research! Spinoff technology proves that it is worthwhile to invest in science research because it could enrich people's lives in unexpected ways.

The first spinoff technology worth mentioning is baby food. In space, where astronauts have limited access to fresh food and fewer options about their daily meals, malnutrition is a serious concern. Consequently, NASA researchers were looking for ways to enhance the nutritional value of astronauts' food. Scientists found that a certain type of algae could be added to food, improving the food's neurological benefits. When experts in the commercial food industry learned of this algae's potential to boost brain health, they were quick to begin their own research. The nutritional substance from algae then developed into a product called life's DHA, which can be found in over 90% of infant food sold in America.

Another intriguing example of a spinoff technology can be found in fashion. People who are always dropping their sunglasses may have invested in a pair of sunglasses with scratch resistant lenses—that is, it's impossible to scratch the glass, even if the glasses are dropped on an abrasive surface. This innovation is incredibly advantageous for people who are clumsy, but most shoppers don't know that this technology was originally developed by NASA. Scientists first created scratch resistant glass to help protect costly and crucial equipment from getting scratched in space, especially the helmet visors in space suits. However, sunglasses companies later realized that this technology could be profitable for their products, and they licensed the technology from NASA.

1. What is the main purpose of this article?
    a. To advise consumers to do more research before making a purchase
    b. To persuade readers to support NASA research
    c. To tell a narrative about the history of space technology
    d. To define and describe instances of spinoff technology

2. What is the organizational structure of this article?
    a. A general definition followed by more specific examples
    b. A general opinion followed by supporting arguments
    c. An important moment in history followed by chronological details
    d. A popular misconception followed by counterevidence

3. Why did NASA scientists research algae?
    a. They already knew algae was healthy for babies.
    b. They were interested in how to grow food in space.
    c. They were looking for ways to add health benefits to food.
    d. They hoped to use it to protect expensive research equipment.

4. What does the word "neurological" mean in the second paragraph?
    a. Related to the body
    b. Related to the brain
    c. Related to vitamins
    d. Related to technology

5. Why does the author mention space suit helmets?
    a. To give an example of astronaut fashion
    b. To explain where sunglasses got their shape
    c. To explain how astronauts protect their eyes
    d. To give an example of valuable space equipment

6. Which statement would the author probably NOT agree with?
    a. Consumers don't always know the history of the products they are buying.
    b. Sometimes new innovations have unexpected applications.
    c. It is difficult to make money from scientific research.
    d. Space equipment is often very expensive.

Questions 7-13 are based on the following passage:

People who argue that William Shakespeare is not responsible for the plays attributed to his name are known as anti-Stratfordians (from the name of Shakespeare's birthplace, Stratford-upon-Avon). The most common anti-Stratfordian claim is that William Shakespeare simply was not educated enough or from a high enough social class to have written plays overflowing with references to such a wide range of subjects like history, the classics, religion, and international culture. William Shakespeare was the son of a glove-maker, he only had a basic grade school education, and he never set foot outside of England—so how could he have produced plays of such sophistication and imagination? How could he have written in such detail about historical figures and events, or about different cultures and locations around Europe? According to anti-Stratfordians, the depth of knowledge contained in Shakespeare's plays suggests a well-traveled writer from a wealthy background with a university education, not a countryside writer like Shakespeare. But in fact, there is not much substance to such speculation, and most anti-Stratfordian arguments can be refuted with a little background about Shakespeare's time and upbringing.

First of all, those who doubt Shakespeare's authorship often point to his common birth and brief education as stumbling blocks to his writerly genius. Although it is true that Shakespeare did not come from a noble class, his father was a very *successful* glove-maker and his mother was from a very wealthy land owning family—so while Shakespeare may have had a country upbringing, he was certainly from a well-off family and would have been educated accordingly. Also, even though he did not attend university, grade school education in Shakespeare's time was actually quite rigorous and exposed students to classic drama through writers like Seneca and Ovid. It is not unreasonable to believe that Shakespeare received a very solid foundation in poetry and literature from his early schooling.

Next, anti-Stratfordians tend to question how Shakespeare could write so extensively about countries and cultures he had never visited before (for instance, several of his most famous works like *Romeo and Juliet* and *The Merchant of Venice* were set in Italy, on the opposite side of Europe!). But again, this criticism does not hold up under scrutiny. For one thing, Shakespeare was living in London, a bustling metropolis of international trade, the most populous city in England, and a political and cultural hub of Europe. In the daily crowds of people, Shakespeare would certainly have been able to meet travelers from other countries and hear firsthand accounts of life in their home country. And, in addition to the influx of information from world travelers, this was also the age of the printing press, a jump in technology that made it possible to print and circulate books much more easily than in the past. This also allowed for a freer flow of information across different countries, allowing people to read about life and ideas from throughout Europe. One needn't travel the continent in order to learn and write about its culture.

7. What is the main purpose of this article?
    a. To explain two sides of an argument and allow readers to choose which side they agree with
    b. To encourage readers to be skeptical about the authorship of famous poems and plays
    c. To give historical background about an important literary figure
    d. To criticize a theory by presenting counterevidence

8. Which sentence contains the author's thesis?
    a. People who argue that William Shakespeare is not responsible for the plays attributed to his name are known as anti-Stratfordians.
    b. But in fact, there is not much substance to such speculation, and most anti-Stratfordian arguments can be refuted with a little background about Shakespeare's time and upbringing.
    c. It is not unreasonable to believe that Shakespeare received a very solid foundation in poetry and literature from his early schooling.
    d. Next, anti-Stratfordians tend to question how Shakespeare could write so extensively about countries and cultures he had never visited before.

9. How does the author respond to the claim that Shakespeare was not well-educated because he did not attend university?
    a. By insisting upon Shakespeare's natural genius
    b. By explaining grade school curriculum in Shakespeare's time
    c. By comparing Shakespeare with other uneducated writers of his time
    d. By pointing out that Shakespeare's wealthy parents probably paid for private tutors

10. What does the word "bustling" in the third paragraph most nearly mean?
    a. Busy
    b. Foreign
    c. Expensive
    d. Undeveloped

11. What can be inferred from the article?
    a. Shakespeare's peers were jealous of his success and wanted to attack his reputation.
    b. Until recently, classic drama was only taught in universities.
    c. International travel was extremely rare in Shakespeare's time.
    d. In Shakespeare's time, glove-makers were not part of the upper class.

12. Why does the author mention *Romeo and Juliet*?
    a. It is Shakespeare's most famous play.
    b. It was inspired by Shakespeare's trip to Italy.
    c. It is an example of a play set outside of England.
    d. It was unpopular when Shakespeare first wrote it.

13. Which statement would the author probably agree with?
   a. It is possible to learn things from reading rather than from firsthand experience.
   b. If you want to be truly cultured, you need to travel the world
   c. People never become successful without a university education.
   d. All of the world's great art comes from Italy.

Questions 14-17 are based on the following passage which is adapted from Abraham Lincoln's Address Delivered at the Dedication of the Cemetery at Gettysburg, November 19, 1863:

Four score and seven years ago our fathers brought forth on this continent, a new nation, conceived in liberty, and dedicated to the proposition that all men are created equal.

Now we are engaged in a great civil war, testing whether that nation, or any nation so conceived and so dedicated, can long endure. We are met on a great battlefield of that war. We have come to dedicate a portion of that field, as a final resting place for those who here gave their lives that this nation might live. It is altogether fitting and proper that we should do this.

But, in a larger sense, we cannot dedicate --- we cannot consecrate that we cannot hallow --- this ground. The brave men, living and dead, who struggled here, have consecrated it, far above our poor power to add or detract. The world will little note, nor long remember what we say here, but it can never forget what they did here. It is for us the living, rather, to be dedicated here to the unfinished work which they who fought here have thus far so nobly advanced. It is rather for us to be here and dedicated to the great task remaining before us--- that from these honored dead we take increased devotion to that cause for which they gave the last full measure of devotion --- that we here highly resolve that these dead shall not have died in vain --- that these this nation, under God, shall have a new birth of freedom--- and that government of people, by the people, for the people, shall not perish from the earth.

14. The best description for the phrase "Four score and seven years ago" is?
   a. A unit of measurement
   b. A period of time
   c. A literary movement
   d. A statement of political reform

15. Which war is Abraham Lincoln referring to in the following passage? "Now we are engaged in a great civil war, testing whether that nation, or any nation so conceived and so dedicated, can long endure."
   a. World War I
   b. The War of Spanish Succession
   c. World War II
   d. The American Civil War

16. What message is the author trying to convey through this address?
   a. The audience should consider the death of the people that fought in the war as an example and perpetuate the ideals of freedom that the soldiers died fighting for.
   b. The audience should honor the dead by establishing an annual memorial service.
   c. The audience should form a militia that would overturn the current political structure.
   d. The audience should forget the lives that were lost and discredit the soldiers.

17. What is the effect of Lincoln's statement in the following passage? "But, in a larger sense, we cannot dedicate --- we cannot consecrate that we cannot hallow --- this ground. The brave men, living and dead, who struggled here, have consecrated it, far above our poor power to add or detract."
    a. His comparison emphasizes the great sacrifice of the soldiers who fought in the war.
    b. His comparison serves as a remainder of the inadequacies of his audience.
    c. His comparison serves as a catalyst for guilt and shame among audience members.
    d. His comparison attempts to illuminate the great differences between soldiers and civilians.

Questions 18-20 are based on the following passage, which is an adaptation of Robert Louis Stevenson's The Strange Case of Dr. Jekyll and Mr. Hyde:

"Did you ever come across a protégé of his—one Hyde?" He asked.

"Hyde?" repeated Lanyon. "No. Never heard of him. Since my time."

That was the amount of information that the lawyer carried back with him to the great, dark bed on which he tossed to and fro until the small hours of the morning began to grow large. It was a night of little ease to his toiling mind, toiling in mere darkness and besieged by questions.

Six o'clock struck on the bells of the church that was so conveniently near to Mr. Utterson's dwelling, and still he was digging at the problem. Hitherto it had touched him on the intellectual side alone; but; but now his imagination also was engaged, or rather enslaved; and as he lay and tossed in the gross darkness of the night in the curtained room, Mr. Enfield's tale went by before his mind in a scroll of lighted pictures. He would be aware of the great field of lamps in a nocturnal city; then of the figure of a man walking swiftly; then of a child running from the doctor's; and then these met, and that human Juggernaut trod the child down and passed on regardless of her screams. Or else he would see a room in a rich house, where his friend lay asleep, dreaming and smiling at his dreams; and then the door of that room would be opened, the curtains of the bed plucked apart, the sleeper recalled, and, lo! There would stand by his side a figure to whom power was given, and even at that dead hour he must rise and do its bidding. The figure in these two phrases haunted the lawyer all night; and if at anytime he dozed over, it was but to see it glide more stealthily through sleeping houses, or move the more swiftly, and still the more smoothly, even to dizziness, through wider labyrinths of lamplighted city, and at every street corner crush a child and leave her screaming. And still the figure had no face by which he might know it; even in his dreams it had no face, or one that baffled him and melted before his eyes; and thus there it was that there sprung up and grew apace in the lawyer's mind a singularly strong, almost an inordinate, curiosity to behold the features of the real Mr. Hyde. If he could but once set eyes on him, he thought the mystery would lighten and perhaps roll altogether away, as was the habit of mysterious things when well examined. He might see a reason for his friend's strange preference or bondage, and even for the startling clauses of the will. And at least it would be a face worth seeing: the face of a man who was without bowels of mercy: a face which had but to show itself to raise up, in the mind of the unimpressionable Enfield, a spirit of enduring hatred.

From that time forward, Mr. Utterson began to haunt the door in the by street of shops. In the morning before office hours, at noon when business was plenty of time scarce, at night under the face of the full city moon, by all lights and at all hours of solitude or concourse, the lawyer was to be found on his chosen post.

"If he be Mr. Hyde," he had thought, "I should be Mr. Seek."

18. What can one infer about the meaning of the word "Juggernaut" from the author's use of it in the passage?
    a. It is an apparition that appears at daybreak.
    b. It scares children.
    c. It is associated with space travel.
    d. Mr. Utterson finds it soothing.

19. What is the definition of the word *haunt* in the following passage?
    From that time forward, Mr. Utterson began to haunt the door in the by street of shops. In the morning before office hours, at noon when business was plenty of time scarce, at night under the face of the full city moon, by all lights and at all hours of solitude or concourse, the lawyer was to be found on his chosen post.

    a. To levitate
    b. To constantly visit
    c. To terrorize
    d. To daunt

20. What can one reasonably conclude from the final comment of this passage?
    "If he be Mr. Hyde," he had thought, "I should be Mr. Seek."

    a. The speaker is considering a name change.
    b. The speaker is experiencing an identity crisis.
    c. The speaker has mistakenly been looking for the wrong person.
    d. The speaker intends to continue to look for Hyde.

Questions 21-25 are based on the following passage, which is adapted from The Ideas of Physics, Third Edition by Douglas C. Giancoli:

The Electric Battery

The events that led to the discovery of the battery are interesting; for not only was this an important discovery, but it also gave rise to a famous scientific debate between Alessandro Volta and Luigi Galvani, eventually involving many others in the scientific world.

In the 1780's, Galvani, a professor at the University of Bologna (thought to be the world's oldest university still in existence), carried out a long series of experiments on the contraction of a frog's leg muscle through electricity produced by a static-electricity machine. In the course of these investigations, Galvani found, much to his surprise, that contraction of the muscle could be produced by other means as well: when a brass hook was pressed into the frog's spinal cord and then hung from an iron railing that also touched the frog, the leg muscles again would contract. Upon further investigation, Galvani found that this strange but important phenomenon occurred for other pairs of metals as well.

Galvani believed that the source of the electric charge was in the frog muscle or nerve itself and the wire merely transmitted the charge to the proper points. When he published his work in 1791, he termed it "animal electricity." Many wondered, including Galvani himself, if he had discovered the long-sought "life-force."

Volta, at the University of Pavia 125 miles away, was at first skeptical of Galvani's results, but at the urging of his colleagues, he soon confirmed and extended those experiments. Volta doubted Galvani's idea of "animal electricity." Instead he came to believe that the source of the electricity was not in the animal, but rather in the contact between the two metals.

During Volta's careful research, he soon realized that a moist conductor, such as a frog muscle or moisture at the contact point of the two dissimilar metals, was necessary if the effect was to occur. He also saw that the contracting frog muscle was a sensitive instrument for detecting electric potential or voltage, in fact more sensitive than the best available electroscopes that he and others had developed. Volta's research showed that certain combinations of metals produced a greater effect than others.

Volta then conceived his greatest contribution to science. Between a disc of zinc and one of silver he placed a piece of cloth or paper soaked in salt solution or dilute acid and piled a "battery" of such couplings, one on top of another; this "pile" or "battery" produced a much increased potential difference. Indeed, when strips of metal connected to the two ends of the pile were brought close, a spark was produced. Volta had designed and built the first battery.

21. Which statement best details the central idea in this passage?
    a. It details the story of how the battery was originally developed.
    b. It delves into the mechanics of battery operated machines.
    c. It defines the far-reaching effects of battery usage throughout the world.
    d. It invites readers to create innovations that make the world more efficient.

22. Which definition most closely relates to the usage of the word "battery" in the passage?
    a. A group of objects that work in tandem to create a unified effect
    b. A log of assessments
    c. A series
    d. A violent encounter

23. Which researcher was ultimately credited with creating "the first battery"?
    a. Galvani
    b. Pavia
    c. Volta
    d. Bologna

24. Which of the statements reflect information that one could reasonably infer based on Volta's scientific contributions concerning batteries?
    a. The researcher died in a state of shame and obscurity.
    b. Others researchers doubted his ability to create the first battery.
    c. The term "voltage" was created to recognize him for his contribution in the production of batteries.
    d. Researchers now use plastic to further technological advances in the field of electrical current conduction.

25. According to the following passage, which statement best describes the contrast between Volta and Galvani's theory concerning "animal electricity"? "Galvani believed that the source of the electric charge was in the frog muscle or nerve itself and the wire merely transmitted the charge to the proper points. When he published his work in 1791, he termed it "animal electricity." Many wondered, including Galvani himself, if he had discovered the long-sought "life-force."

Volta, at the University of Pavia 125 miles away, was at first skeptical of Galvani's results, but at the urging of his colleagues, he soon confirmed and extended those experiments. Volta doubted Galvani's idea of "animal electricity." Instead he came to believe that the source of the electricity was not in the animal, but rather in the contact between the two metals."

    a. Galvani believed that only frogs were capable of serving as conductors for electricity.
    b. Volta doubted that animals possessed the intellect necessary to properly direct electricity to the proper source.
    c. Galvani believed that animals were carriers of the "life-force" necessary to conduct electricity while Volta felt that the meeting of metals was the catalyst for animal movement in the experiment.
    d. Both researchers held fast to the belief that their theories were the foremost and premiere research in the field.

Questions 26-29 are based upon the following passage, which is an adaptation from Mineralogy --- Encyclopedia International, Grolier

Mineralogy is the science of minerals, which are the naturally occurring elements and compounds that make up the solid parts of the universe. Mineralogy is usually considered in terms of materials in the Earth, but meteorites provide samples of minerals from outside the Earth.

A mineral may be defined as a naturally occurring, homogeneous solid, inorganically formed, with a definite chemical composition and an ordered atomic arrangement. The qualification *naturally occurring* is essential because it is possible to reproduce most minerals in the laboratory. For example, evaporating a solution of sodium chloride produces crystal indistinguishable from those of the mineral halite, but such laboratory-produced crystals are not minerals.

A *homogeneous solid* is one consisting of a single kind of material that cannot be separated into simpler compounds by any physical method. The requirement that a mineral be solid eliminates gases and liquids from consideration. Thus ice is a mineral (a very common one, especially at high altitudes and latitudes) but water is not. Some mineralogists dispute this restriction and would consider both water and native mercury (also a liquid) as minerals.

The restriction of minerals to *inorganically formed* substances eliminates those homogenous solids produced by animals and plants. Thus the shell of an oyster and the pearl inside, though both consist of calcium carbonate indistinguishable chemically or physically from the mineral aragonite comma are not usually considered minerals.

The requirement of a *definite chemical composition* implies that a mineral is a chemical compound, and the composition of a chemical compound is readily expressed by a formula. Mineral formulas may be simple or complex, depending upon the number of elements present and the proportions in which they are combined.

Minerals are crystalline solids, and the presence of an *ordered atomic arrangement* is the criterion of the crystalline state. Under favorable conditions of formation the ordered atomic arrangement is expressed in the external crystal form. In fact, the presence of an ordered atomic arrangement and crystalline solids was deduced from the external regularity of crystals by a French mineralogist, Abbé R. Haüy, early in the 19th century.

26. According to the text, an object or substance must have all of the following criteria to be considered a mineral except for?
    a. Be naturally occurring
    b. Be a homogeneous solid
    c. Be organically formed
    d. Have a definite chemical composition

27. One can deduce that French mineralogist Abbé R. Haüy specialized in what field of study?
    a. Geology
    b. Psychology
    c. Biology
    d. Botany

28. What is the definition of the word "homogeneous" as it appears in the following passage?

"A homogeneous solid is one consisting of a single kind of material that cannot be separated into simpler compounds by any physical method."
    a. Made of similar substances
    b. Differing in some areas
    c. Having a higher atomic mass
    d. Lacking necessary properties

29. The suffix -logy refers to:
    a. The properties of
    b. The chemical makeup of
    c. The study of
    d. The classification of

Questions 30-33 are based upon the following passage:

This excerpt is adaptation from *Our Vanishing Wildlife,* by William T. Hornaday

> Three years ago, I think there were not many bird-lovers in the United States, who believed it possible to prevent the total extinction of both egrets from our fauna. All the known rookeries accessible to plume-hunters had been totally destroyed. Two years ago, the secret discovery of several small, hidden colonies prompted William Dutcher, President of the National Association of Audubon Societies, and Mr. T. Gilbert Pearson, Secretary, to attempt the protection of those colonies. With a fund contributed for the purpose, wardens were hired and duly commissioned. As previously stated, one of those wardens was shot dead in cold blood by a plume hunter. The task of guarding swamp rookeries from the attacks of money-hungry desperadoes to whom the accursed plumes were worth their weight in gold, is a very chancy proceeding. There is now one warden in Florida who says that "before they get my rookery they will first have to get me."
>
> Thus far the protective work of the Audubon Association has been successful. Now there are twenty colonies, which contain all told, about 5,000 egrets and about 120,000 herons and ibises which are guarded by the Audubon wardens. One of the most

important is on Bird Island, a mile out in Orange Lake, central Florida, and it is ably defended by Oscar E. Baynard. To-day, the plume hunters who do not dare to raid the guarded rookeries are trying to study out the lines of flight of the birds, to and from their feeding-grounds, and shoot them in transit. Their motto is—"Anything to beat the law, and get the plumes." It is there that the state of Florida should take part in the war.

The success of this campaign is attested by the fact that last year a number of egrets were seen in eastern Massachusetts—for the first time in many years. And so to-day the question is, can the wardens continue to hold the plume-hunters at bay?

30. What is the meaning of the word *rookeries* in the following text?
    To-day, the plume hunters who do not dare to raid the guarded rookeries are trying to study out the lines of flight of the birds, to and from their feeding-grounds, and shoot them in transit.

    a. Houses in a slum area
    b. A place where hunters gather to trade tools
    c. A place where wardens go to trade stories
    d. A colony of breeding birds

31. What is on Bird Island?
    a. Hunters selling plumes
    b. An important bird colony
    c. Bird Island Battle between the hunters and the wardens
    d. An important egret with unique plumes

32. What is the main purpose of the passage?
    a. To persuade the audience to act in preservation of the bird colonies
    b. To show the effect hunting egrets has had on the environment
    c. To argue that the preservation of bird colonies has had a negative impact on the environment.
    d. To demonstrate the success of the protective work of the Audubon Association

33. Why are hunters trying to study the lines of flight of the birds?
    a. To study ornithology, one must know the lines of flight that birds take.
    b. To help wardens preserve the lives of the birds
    c. To have a better opportunity to hunt the birds
    d. To builds their homes under the lines of flight because they believe it brings good luck

Questions 34-39 are based upon the following passage:

The Myth of Head Heat Loss

It has recently been brought to my attention that most people believe that 75% of your body heat is lost through your head. I had certainly heard this before, and am not going to attempt to say I didn't believe it when I first heard it. It is natural to be gullible to anything said with enough authority. But the "fact" that the majority of your body heat is lost through your head is a lie.

Let me explain. Heat loss is proportional to surface area exposed. An elephant loses a great deal more heat than an anteater, because it has a much greater surface area than an anteater. Each cell has mitochondria that produce energy in the form of heat, and it takes a lot more energy to run an elephant than an anteater.

So, each part of your body loses its proportional amount of heat in accordance with its surface area. The human torso probably loses the most heat, though the legs lose a significant amount as well. Some people have asked, "Why does it feel so much warmer when you cover your head than when you don't?" Well, that's because your head, because it is not clothed, is losing a lot of heat while the clothing on the rest of your body provides insulation. If you went outside with a hat and pants but no shirt, not only would you look stupid but your heat loss would be significantly greater because so much more of you would be exposed. So, if given the choice to cover your chest or your head in the cold, choose the chest. It could save your life.

34. What is the primary purpose of this passage?
    a. To provide evidence that disproves a myth
    b. To compare elephants and anteaters
    c. To explain why it is appropriate to wear clothes in winter
    d. To show how people are gullible

35. Which of the following best describes the main idea of the passage?
    a. It is better to wear a shirt than a hat
    b. Heat loss is proportional to surface area exposed
    c. It is natural to be gullible
    d. The human chest loses the most heat

36. Why does the author compare elephants and anteaters?
    a. To express an opinion
    b. To give an example that helps clarify the main point
    c. To show the differences between them
    d. To persuade why one is better than the other

37. The statement, "If you went outside with a hat and pants but no shirt, not only would you look stupid but your heat loss would be significantly greater because so much more of you would be exposed" is which of the following?
    a. An opinion
    b. A fact
    c. An opinion within a fact
    d. Neither

38. Which of the following best describes the tone of the passage?
    a. Harsh
    b. Angry
    c. Casual
    d. Indifferent

39. Which of the following sentences provides the best evidence to support the main idea?
    a. "It is natural to be gullible to anything said with enough authority."
    b. "Each part of your body loses its proportional amount of heat in accordance with its surface area."
    c. "If given the choice to cover your chest or your head in the cold, choose the chest."
    d. "But the 'fact' that the majority of your body heat it lost through your head is a lie."

Questions 40-47 are based upon the following passage:

The Global Water Crisis

For decades, the world's water supply has been decreasing. At least ten percent of the world population, or over 780 million people, do not have access to potable water. They have to walk for miles, carrying heavy buckets in intense heat in order to obtain the essential life source that comes freely from our faucets.

We are in a global water crisis. Only 2.5% of the water on Earth is suitable for drinking, and over seventy percent of this water is frozen in the polar ice caps, while much of the rest is located deep underground. This leaves a very small percentage available for drinking, yet we see millions of gallons of water wasted on watering huge lawns in deserts like Arizona, or on running dishwashers that are only half-full, or on filling all the personal pools in Los Angeles, meanwhile people in Africa are dying of thirst.

In order to reduce water waste, Americans and citizens of other first world countries should adhere to the following guidelines: run the dishwasher only when it is full, do only full loads of laundry, wash the car with a bucket and not with a hose, take showers only when necessary, swim in public pools, and just be <u>cognizant </u>of how much water they are using in general. Our planet is getting thirstier by the year, and if we do not solve this problem, our species will surely perish.

40. Which of the following best supports the assertion that we need to limit our water usage?
    a. People are wasting water on superfluous things.
    b. There is very little water on earth suitable for drinking.
    c. At least ten percent of the world population does not have access to drinking water.
    d. There is plenty of drinking water in first world countries, but not anywhere else.

41. How is the content in the selection organized?
    a. In chronological order
    b. Compare and contrast
    c. As a set of problems and solutions
    d. As a series of descriptions

42. Which of the following, if true, would challenge the assertion that we are in a global water crisis?
    a. There are abundant water stores on earth that scientists are not reporting.
    b. Much of the water we drink comes from rain.
    c. People in Africa only have to walk less than a mile to get water.
    d. Most Americans only run the dishwasher when it is full.

43. The selection is written in which of the following styles?
    a. As a narrative
    b. In a persuasive manner
    c. As an informative piece
    d. As a series of descriptions

44. Which of the following is implicitly stated within the following sentence? "This leaves a very small percentage available for drinking, yet we see millions of gallons of water wasted on watering huge lawns in deserts like Arizona, or on running dishwashers that are only half-full, or on filling all the personal pools in Los Angeles, meanwhile people in Africa are dying of thirst."
    a. People run dishwashers that are not full.
    b. People in Africa are dying of thirst.
    c. People take water for granted.
    d. People should stop watering their lawns.

45. Why does the author mention that people have to walk for miles in intense heat to get water?
    a. To inform the reader on the hardships of living in a third world country.
    b. To inspire compassion in the reader.
    c. To show that water is only available in first world countries.
    d. To persuade the reader to reduce their water usage.

46. What is meant by the word <u>cognizant</u>?
    a. To be interested
    b. To be amused
    c. To be mindful
    d. To be accepting

47. What is the main idea of the passage?
    a. People should reduce their water usage.
    b. There is very little drinking water on earth.
    c. People take their access to water for granted.
    d. People should swim in public pools.

Directions for questions 48–55: Read the statement or passage and then choose the best answer to the question. Answer the question based on what is stated or implied in the statement or passage.

48. There are two major kinds of cameras on the market right now for amateur photographers. Camera enthusiasts can either purchase a digital single-lens reflex camera (DSLR) camera or a compact system camera (CSC). The main difference between a DSLR and a CSC is that the DSLR has a full-sized sensor, which means it fits in a much larger body. The CSC uses a mirrorless system, which makes for a lighter, smaller camera. While both take quality pictures, the DSLR generally has better picture quality due to the larger sensor. CSCs still take very good quality pictures and are more convenient to carry than a DSLR. This makes the CSC an ideal choice for the amateur photographer looking to step up from a point-and-shoot camera.

What is the main difference between the DSLR and CSC?
    a. The picture quality is better in the DSLR.
    b. The CSC is less expensive than the DSLR.
    c. The DSLR is a better choice for amateur photographers.
    d. The DSLR's larger sensor makes it a bigger camera than the CSC.

49. When selecting a career path, it's important to explore the various options available. Many students entering college may shy away from a major because they don't know much about it. For example, many students won't opt for a career as an actuary, because they aren't exactly sure what it entails. They would be missing out on a career that is very lucrative and in high demand. Actuaries work in the insurance field and assess risks and premiums. The average salary of an actuary is $100,000 per year. Another career option students may avoid, due to lack of knowledge of the field, is a hospitalist. This is a physician that specializes in the care of patients in a hospital, as opposed to those seen in private practices. The average salary of a hospitalist is upwards of $200,000. It pays to do some digging and find out more about these lesser-known career fields.

What is an actuary?
    a. A doctor who works in a hospital.
    b. The same as a hospitalist.
    c. An insurance agent who works in a hospital.
    d. A person who assesses insurance risks and premiums.

50. Hard water occurs when rainwater mixes with minerals from rock and soil. Hard water has a high mineral count, including calcium and magnesium. The mineral deposits from hard water can stain hard surfaces in bathrooms and kitchens as well as clog pipes. Hard water can stain dishes, ruin clothes, and reduce the life of any appliances it touches, such as hot water heaters, washing machines, and humidifiers.

One solution is to install a water softener to reduce the mineral content of water, but this can be costly. Running vinegar through pipes and appliances and using vinegar to clean hard surfaces can also help with mineral deposits.

From this passage, what can be concluded?
    a. Hard water can cause a lot of problems for homeowners.
    b. Calcium is good for pipes and hard surfaces.
    c. Water softeners are easy to install.
    d. Vinegar is the only solution to hard water problems.

51. Coaches of kids' sports teams are increasingly concerned about the behavior of parents at games. Parents are screaming and cursing at coaches, officials, players, and other parents. Physical fights have even broken out at games. Parents need to be reminded that coaches are volunteers, giving up their time and energy to help kids develop in their chosen sport. The goal of kids' sports teams is to learn and develop skills, but it's also to have fun. When parents are out of control at games and practices, it takes the fun out of the sport.

From this passage, what can be concluded?
    a. Coaches are modeling good behavior for kids.
    b. Organized sports are not good for kids.
    c. Parents' behavior at their kids' games needs to change.
    d. Parents and coaches need to work together.

52. While scientists aren't entirely certain why tornadoes form, they have some clues into the process. Tornadoes are dangerous funnel clouds that occur during a large thunderstorm. When warm, humid air near the ground meets cold, dry air from above, a column of the warm air can be drawn up into the clouds. Winds at different altitudes blowing at different speeds make the column of air rotate. As the spinning column of air picks up speed, a funnel cloud is formed. This funnel cloud moves rapidly and haphazardly. Rain and hail inside the cloud cause it to touch down, creating a tornado. Tornadoes move in a rapid and unpredictable pattern, making them extremely destructive and dangerous. Scientists continue to study tornadoes to improve radar detection and warning times.

The main purpose of this passage is to do which of the following?
    a. Show why tornadoes are dangerous.
    b. Explain how a tornado forms.
    c. Compare thunderstorms to tornadoes.
    d. Explain what to do in the event of a tornado.

53. Many people are unsure of exactly how the digestive system works. Digestion begins in the mouth where teeth grind up food and saliva break it down, making it easier for the body to absorb. Next, the food moves to the esophagus, and it is pushed into the stomach. The stomach is where food is stored and broken down further by acids and digestive enzymes, preparing it for passage into the intestines. The small intestine is where the nutrients are taken from food and passed into the blood stream. Other essential organs like the liver, gall bladder, and pancreas aid the stomach in breaking down food and absorbing nutrients. Finally, food waste is passed into the large intestine where it is eliminated by the body.

The purpose of this passage is to do which of the following?
    a. Explain how the liver works.
    b. Show why it is important to eat healthy foods.
    c. Explain how the digestive system works.
    d. Show how nutrients are absorbed by the small intestine.

54. Osteoporosis is a medical condition that occurs when the body loses bone or makes too little bone. This can lead to brittle, fragile bones that easily break. Bones are already porous, and when osteoporosis sets in, the spaces in bones become much larger, causing them to weaken. Both men and women can contract osteoporosis, though it is most common in women over age 50. Loss of bone can be silent and progressive, so it is important to be proactive in prevention of the disease.

The main purpose of this passage is to do which of the following?
    a. Discuss some of the ways people contract osteoporosis.
    b. Describe different treatment options for those with osteoporosis.
    c. Explain how to prevent osteoporosis.
    d. Define osteoporosis.

55. Vacationers looking for a perfect experience should opt out of Disney parks and try a trip on Disney Cruise Lines. While a park offers rides, characters, and show experiences, it also includes long lines, often very hot weather, and enormous crowds. A Disney Cruise, on the other hand, is a relaxing, luxurious vacation that includes many of the same experiences as the parks, minus the crowds and lines. The cruise has top-notch food, maid service, water slides, multiple pools, Broadway-quality shows, and daily character experiences for kids. There are also many activities, such as bingo, trivia contests, and dance parties that can entertain guests of all ages. The cruise even stops at Disney's private island for a beach barbecue with characters, waterslides, and water sports. Those looking for the Disney experience without the hassle should book a Disney cruise.

The main purpose of this passage is to do which of the following?
    a. Explain how to book a Disney cruise.
    b. Show what Disney parks have to offer.
    c. Show why Disney parks are expensive.
    d. Compare Disney parks to the Disney cruise.

Answer Explanations

1. D: To define and describe instances of spinoff technology. This is an example of a purpose question—*why* did the author write this? The article contains facts, definitions, and other objective information without telling a story or arguing an opinion. In this case, the purpose of the article is to inform the reader. The only answer choice that is related to giving information is answer Choice *D*: to define and describe.

2. A: A general definition followed by more specific examples. This organization question asks readers to analyze the structure of the essay. The topic of the essay is about spinoff technology; the first paragraph gives a general definition of the concept, while the following two paragraphs offer more detailed examples to help illustrate this idea.

3. C: They were looking for ways to add health benefits to food. This reading comprehension question can be answered based on the second paragraph—scientists were concerned about astronauts' nutrition and began researching useful nutritional supplements. A in particular is not true because it reverses the order of discovery (first NASA identified algae for astronaut use, and then it was further developed for use in baby food).

4. B: Related to the brain. This vocabulary question could be answered based on the reader's prior knowledge; but even for readers who have never encountered the word "neurological" before, the passage does provide context clues. The very next sentence talks about "this algae's potential to boost brain health," which is a paraphrase of "neurological benefits." From this context, readers should be able to infer that "neurological" is related to the brain.

5. D: To give an example of valuable space equipment. This purpose question requires readers to understand the relevance of the given detail. In this case, the author mentions "costly and crucial equipment" before mentioning space suit visors, which are given as an example of something that is very valuable. *A* is not correct because fashion is only related to sunglasses, not to NASA equipment. *B* can be eliminated because it is simply not mentioned in the passage. While *C* seems like it could be a true statement, it is also not relevant to what is being explained by the author.

6. C: It is difficult to make money from scientific research. The article gives several examples of how businesses have been able to capitalize on NASA research, so it is unlikely that the author would agree with this statement. Evidence for the other answer choices can be found in the article: *A*, the author mentions that "many consumers are unaware that products they are buying are based on NASA research"; *B* is a general definition of spinoff technology; and *D* is mentioned in the final paragraph.

7. D: To criticize a theory by presenting counterevidence. The author mentions anti-Stratfordian arguments in the first paragraph, but then goes on to debunk these theories with more facts about Shakespeare's life in the second and third paragraphs. *A* is not correct because, while the author does present arguments from both sides, the author is far from unbiased; in fact, the author clearly disagrees with anti-Stratfordians. *B* is also not correct because it is more closely aligned to the beliefs of anti-Stratfordians, whom the author disagrees with. *C* can be eliminated because, while it is true that the author gives historical background, the main purpose of the article is using that information to disprove a theory.

8. B: But in fact, there is not much substance to such speculation, and most anti-Stratfordian arguments can be refuted with a little background about Shakespeare's time and upbringing. The thesis is a statement that contains the author's topic and main idea. As seen in question 7, the main purpose of this article is to use historical evidence to provide counterarguments to anti-Stratfordians. *A* is simply a definition; *C* is a supporting detail, not a main idea; and *D* represents an idea of anti-Stratfordians, not the author's opinion.

9. B: By explaining grade school curriculum in Shakespeare's time. This question asks readers to refer to the organizational structure of the article and demonstrate understanding of how the author provides details to support their argument. This particular detail can be found in the second paragraph: "even though he did not attend university, grade school education in Shakespeare's time was actually quite rigorous."

10. A: Busy. This is a vocabulary question that can be answered using context clues. Other sentences in the paragraph describe London as "the most populous city in England" filled with "crowds of people," giving an image of a busy city full of people. *B* is not correct because London was in Shakespeare's home country, not a foreign one. *C* is not mentioned in the passage. *D* is not a good answer choice because the passage describes how London was a popular and important city, probably not an underdeveloped one.

11. D: In Shakespeare's time, glove-makers were not part of the upper class. Anti-Stratfordians doubt Shakespeare's ability because he was not from the upper class; his father was a glove-maker; therefore, in at least this instance, glove-makers were not included in the upper class (this is an example of inductive reasoning, or using two specific pieces of information to draw a more general conclusion).

12. C: It is an example of a play set outside of England. This detail comes from the third paragraph, where the author responds to skeptics who claim that Shakespeare wrote too much about places he never visited, so *Romeo and Juliet* is mentioned as a famous example of a play with a foreign setting. In order to answer this question, readers need to understand the author's main purpose in the third paragraph and how the author uses details to support this purpose. *A* and *D* are not mentioned in the passage, and *B* is clearly not true because the passage mentions more than once that Shakespeare never left England.

13. A: It is possible to learn things from reading rather than from firsthand experience. This inference can be made from the final paragraph, where the author refutes anti-Stratfordian skepticism by pointing out that books about life in Europe could easily circulate throughout London. From this statement, readers can conclude that the author believes it is possible that Shakespeare learned about European culture from books, rather than visiting the continent on his own. *B* is not true because the author believes that Shakespeare contributed to English literature without traveling extensively. Similarly, *C* is not a good answer because the author explains how Shakespeare got his education without university. *D* can also be eliminated because the author describes Shakespeare's genius and clearly Shakespeare is not from Italy.

14. B: A period of time. "Four score and seven years ago" is the equivalent of eighty-seven years, because the word "score" means "twenty." *A* and *C* are incorrect because the context for describing a unit of measurement or a literary movement is lacking. *D* is incorrect because although Lincoln's speech is a cornerstone in political rhetoric, the phrase "Four score and seven years ago" is better narrowed to a period of time.

15. D: Abraham Lincoln is the former president of the United States, so the correct answer is *D*, "The American Civil War." Though the U.S. was involved in World War I and II, *A* and *C* are incorrect because a civil war specifically means citizens fighting within the same country. *B* is incorrect, as "The War of Spanish Succession" involved Spain, Italy, Germany, and Holland, and not the United States.

16. A: The speech calls on the audience to consider the soldiers who died on the battlefield as ideas to perpetuate freedom so that their deaths would not be in vain. *B* is incorrect because, although they are there to "dedicate a portion of that field," there is no mention in the text of an annual memorial service. *C* is incorrect because there is no charged language in the text, only reverence for the dead. *D* is incorrect because "forget[ting] the lives that were lost" is the opposite of what Lincoln is suggesting.

17. A: Choice *A* is correct because Lincoln's intention was to memorialize the soldiers who had fallen as a result of war as well as celebrate those who had put their lives in danger for the sake of their country. Choices *B, C,* and *D* are incorrect because Lincoln's speech was supposed to foster a sense of pride among the members of the audience while connecting them to the soldiers' experiences, not to alienate or discourage them.

18. B: It scares children. The passage states that the Juggernaut causes the children to scream. Choices *A* and *D* don't apply because the text doesn't mention either of these instances specifically. Choice *C* is incorrect because there is nothing in the text that mentions space travel.

19. B: To constantly visit. The mention of *morning, noon,* and *night* make it clear that the word *haunt* refers to frequent appearances at various locations. Choice *A* doesn't work because the text makes no mention of levitating. Choices *C* and *D* are not correct because the text makes mention of Mr. Utterson's anguish and disheartenment because of his failure to find Hyde but does not make mention of Mr. Utterson's feelings negatively affecting anyone else.

20. D: The speaker intends to continue to look for Hyde. Choices *A* and *B* are not possible answers because the text doesn't refer to any name changes or an identity crisis, despite Mr. Utterson's extreme obsession with finding Hyde. The text also makes no mention of a mistaken identity when referring to Hyde, so Choice *C* is also incorrect.

21. A: The story is dedicated to telling about the origin of the battery. It doesn't explicitly explain the mechanics of battery operated machines or the far-reaching effects of battery usage, like Choices *B* and *C* suggest. Choice *D* also doesn't work because it does not explicitly encourage readers to take part in new innovations.

22. A: Choices *B* and *D* are incorrect because the text makes no mention of an assessment or a violent encounter. Choice *C* is a possibility; however, Choice *A* is the correct answer because Volta placed things in a particular order to achieve a given result.

23. C: The text states that Volta is credited with creating the first battery. Choice *A*, Galvani, had a part in the discovery of the battery because Volta built upon Galvani's previous research. Choice *B*, Pavia, is the university that Volta attended. Choice *D*, Bologna, is the name of the university that Galvani attended.

24. C: The text supports the idea that the term "voltage" has a direct correlation to the fact that Volta is the scientist credited with originally developing batteries. *A* is incorrect because the text does not explain how the researcher died, or that he had failed in any way. *B* is incorrect because information about the researcher's peers is not represented in the text. *D* is incorrect because the text does not divulge the advances of modern researchers.

25. C: The text corroborates the assertion concerning Galvani's belief about the role of animals' life-force in inducing muscle movements. Volta's initial doubt in Galvani's belief led Volta to further the research Galvani had started. *A* is incorrect because it leaves out any information concerning Volta. *B* is incorrect because Volta was not concerned with the intellect of the animals, but rather their ability to contain the "life-force" of electricity. D is incorrect because the text does not depict either researcher believing their own theories were the foremost research in the field.

26. C: The text mentions all of the listed properties of minerals except the instance of minerals being organically formed. Objects or substances must be naturally occurring, must be a homogeneous solid, and must have a definite chemical composition in order to be considered a mineral.

27. A: Choice A is the correct answer because geology is the study of earth related science. Choice B is incorrect because psychology is the study of the mind and behavior. Choice C is incorrect because biology is the study of life and living organisms. Choice D is incorrect because botany is the study of plants.

28. A: Choice A is the correct answer because the prefix "homo" means same. Choice B is incorrect because "differing in some areas" would be linked to the root word "hetero," meaning "different" or "other."

29: C: Choice C is the correct answer because *-logy* refers to the study of a particular subject matter.

30. D: A *rookery* is a colony of breeding birds. Although *rookery* could mean Choice A, houses in a slum area, it does not make sense in this context. Choices B and C are both incorrect, as this is not a place for hunters to trade tools or for wardens to trade stories.

31. B: An important bird colony. The previous sentence is describing "twenty colonies" of birds, so what follows should be a bird colony. Choice A may be true, but we have no evidence of this in the text. Choice C does touch on the tension between the hunters and wardens, but there is no official "Bird Island Battle" mentioned in the text. Choice D does not exist in the text.

32. D: To demonstrate the success of the protective work of the Audubon Association. The text mentions several different times how and why the association has been successful and gives examples to back this fact. Choice A is incorrect because although the article, in some instances, calls certain people to act, it is not the purpose of the entire passage. There is no way to tell if Choices B and C are correct, as they are not mentioned in the text.

33. C: To have a better opportunity to hunt the birds. Choice A might be true in a general sense, but it is not relevant to the context of the text. Choice B is incorrect because the hunters are not studying lines of flight to help wardens, but to hunt birds. Choice D is incorrect because nothing in the text mentions that hunters are trying to build homes underneath lines of flight of birds for good luck.

34. A: Not only does the article provide examples to disprove a myth, the title also suggests that the article is trying to disprove a myth. Further, the sentence, "But the 'fact' that the majority of your body heat is lost through your head is a lie," and then the subsequent "let me explain," demonstrates the author's intention in disproving a myth. B is incorrect because although the selection does compare elephants and anteaters, it does so in order to prove a point, and is not the primary reason that the selection was written. C is incorrect because even though the article mentions somebody wearing clothes in the winter, and that doing so could save your life, wearing clothes in the winter is not the primary reason this article was written. D is incorrect because the article only mentions that people are gullible once, and makes no further comment on the matter, so this cannot be the primary purpose.

35. B: If the myth is that most of one's body heat is lost through their head, then the fact that heat loss is proportional to surface area exposed is the best evidence that disproves it, since one's head is a great deal less surface area than the rest of the body, making *B* the correct choice. "It is better to wear a shirt than a hat" does not provide evidence that disproves the fact that the head loses more heat than the rest of the body. Thus, *A* is incorrect. *C* is incorrect because gullibility is mentioned only once in this passage and the rest of the article ignores this statement, so clearly it is not the main idea. Finally, *D* is incorrect because though the article mentions that the human chest probably loses the most heat, it is to provide an example of the evidence that heat loss is proportional to surface area exposed, so this is not the main idea of the passage.

36. B: Choice *B* is correct because the author is trying to demonstrate the main idea, which is that heat loss is proportional to surface area, and so they compare two animals with different surface areas to clarify the main point. *A* is incorrect because the author uses elephants and anteaters to prove a point, that heat loss is proportional to surface area, not to express an opinion. *C* is incorrect because though the author does use them to show differences, they do so in order to give examples that prove the above points, so *C* is not the best answer. *D* is incorrect because there is no language to indicate favoritism between the two animals.

37. C: Since there is an opinion presented along with a fact, *C* is the correct answer. *A* is incorrect—"Not only would you look stupid," is an opinion because there is no way to prove that somebody would look stupid by not wearing a shirt in the cold, even if that may be a popular opinion. However, this opinion is sandwiched inside a factual statement. *B* is incorrect because again, this is a factual statement, but it has been editorialized by interjecting an opinion. Because of the presence of both a fact and an opinion, *D* is the opposite of the correct answer.

38. C: Because of the way that the author addresses the reader, and also the colloquial language that the author uses (i.e., "let me explain," "so," "well," didn't," "you would look stupid," etc.), *C* is the best answer because it has a much more casual tone than the usual informative article. Choice *A* may be a tempting choice because the author says the "fact" that most of one's heat is lost through their head is a "lie," and that someone who does not wear a shirt in the cold looks stupid, but it only happens twice within all the diction of the passage and it does not give an overall tone of harshness. *B* is incorrect because again, while not necessarily nice, the language does not carry an angry charge. The author is clearly not indifferent to the subject because of the passionate language that they use, so *D* is incorrect.

39. B: Choice *B* is correct because since the primary purpose of the article is to provide evidence to disprove the myth that most of a person's heat is lost through their head, then each part of the body losing heat in proportion to its surface area is the best evidence to disprove the myth. *A* is incorrect because again, gullibility is not a main contributor to this article, but it may be common to see questions on the test that give the same wrong answer in order to try and trick the test taker. Choice *C* only suggests what you should do with this information; it is not the primary evidence itself. Choice *D,* while tempting, is actually not evidence. It does not give any reason for why it is a lie; it simply states that it is. Evidence is factual information that supports a claim.

40. B: Choice *B* is correct because having very little drinking water on earth is a very good reason that one should limit their water usage so that the human population does not run out of drinking water and die out. People wasting water on superfluous things does not support the fact that we need to limit our water usage. It merely states that people are wasteful. Therefore, *A* is incorrect. Answer Choice *C* may be tempting, but it is not the correct one, as this article is not about reducing water usage in order to help those who don't have easy access to water, but about the fact that the planet is running out of drinking water. Choice *D* is incorrect because nowhere in the article does it state that only first world countries have access to drinking water.

41. C: The primary purpose is to present a problem (the planet is running out of water) with a solution (to reduce water waste), therefore the correct answer is *C*. Choice *A* is incorrect because the passage does not have a sequential timeline of events and is therefore not in chronological order. It may be tempting to think the author compares and contrasts people who do not have access to drinking water to those who do, but that does not fit with the primary purpose of the article, which is to co nvince people to reduce their water usage. Thus, Choice *B* is incorrect. Choice *D* is incorrect because descriptions are not the primary content of this article. Remember that a descriptive writing style describes people, settings, or situations in great detail with many adjectives. While a descriptive writing voice may be used alongside a persuasive writing style, it is generally not the primary voice when trying to convince a reader to take a certain stance.

42. A: If the assertion is that the earth does not have enough drinking water, then having abundant water stores that are not being reported would certainly challenge this assertion. Choice *B* is incorrect because even if much of the water we drink does come from rain, that means the human population would be dependent on rain in order to survive, which would more support the assertion than challenge it. Because the primary purpose of the passage is not to help those who cannot get water, then Choice *C* is not the correct answer. Even if Choice *D* were true, it does not dismiss the other ways in which people are wasteful with water, and is also not the point.

43. B: Choice *B* is correct because the article uses a lot of emotionally charged language and also suggests what needs to be done with the information provided. The article does not contain elements of a narrative, which include plot, setting, characters, and themes. Not only does the article lack these things, but it does not follow a timeline, which is a key element of a narrative voice. Thus, Choice *A* is incorrect. Choice *C* is incorrect because the article uses information in order to be persuasive, but the purpose is not solely to inform on the issue. Choice *D* is incorrect because the article is not written in primarily descriptive language.

44. C: Choice *C* is correct because people who waste water on lawns in the desert, or run a half-full dishwasher, or fill their personal pools are not taking into account how much water they are using because they get an unlimited supply, therefore they are taking it for granted. Choice *A* is incorrect because it is explicitly stated within the text: "running dishwashers that are only half full." Choice *B* is also explicitly stated: "meanwhile people in Africa are dying of thirst." While Choice *D* is implicitly stated within the whole article, it is not implicitly stated within the sentence.

45. B: Choice *B* is correct because the author uses this example in order to show people, through emotional appeal, that they take water for granted, because they get water freely from their faucets, while millions of people have to endure great hardships to get drinking water. Choice *A* does not pertain directly to the main idea of the article, nor does it pertain to the author's purpose. The main idea is that people should reduce their water usage, and the author's purpose is to persuade the reader to do so. A person walking for miles in intense heat does not align with the main point. Choice *C* is incorrect because the selection never mentions that water is only available in first world countries. Choice *D* is the author's purpose for the entire passage, but not the purpose for mentioning the difficulty in getting water for some of the population.

46. C: To be mindful means to be aware, so *C* is the best answer. Choice *A* may be a tempting answer, because if people are interested in the water they are using, they may be more aware of it, but this is not the best answer of the choices. Being amused by water does not make sense in this context, so Choice *B* is incorrect. Being accepting of the amounts of water they use is the opposite of what the author is trying to get the reader to do. Thus, Choice *D* is incorrect.

47. A: The primary purpose and the main idea are essentially the same thing, and the main idea is that people should reduce their water usage because there is not a lot of available drinking water on Earth. Choice *B* is a *reason* that people should reduce their water usage, but it is not the main idea. Choice *C* is a demonstration of how people are not aware of the amount of water they use, but again, not the main idea. Choice *D* is a suggestion for reducing water usage, but still not the main idea.

48. D: The passage directly states that the larger sensor is the main difference between the two cameras. Choices *A* and *B* may be true, but these answers do not identify the major difference between the two cameras. Choice *C* states the opposite of what the paragraph suggests is the best option for amateur photographers, so it is incorrect.

49. D: An actuary assesses risks and sets insurance premiums. While an actuary does work in insurance, the passage does not suggest that actuaries have any affiliation with hospitalists or working in a hospital, so all other choices are incorrect.

50. A: The passage focuses mainly on the problems of hard water. Choice *B* is incorrect because calcium is not good for pipes and hard surfaces. The passage does not say anything about whether water softeners are easy to install, so Choice *C* is incorrect. Choice *D* is also incorrect because the passage does offer other solutions besides vinegar.

51. C: The main point of this paragraph is that parents need to change their poor behavior at their kids' sporting events. Choice *A* is incorrect because the coaches' behavior is not mentioned in the paragraph. Choice *B* suggests that sports are bad for kids, when the paragraph is about parents' behavior, so it is incorrect. While Choice *D* may be true, it offers a specific solution to the problem, which the paragraph does not discuss.

52. B: The main point of this passage is to show how a tornado forms. Choice *A* is off base because while the passage does mention that tornadoes are dangerous, it is not the main focus of the passage. While thunderstorms are mentioned, they are not compared to tornadoes, so Choice *C* is incorrect. Choice *D* is incorrect because the passage does not discuss what to do in the event of a tornado.

53. C: The purpose of this passage is to explain how the digestive system works. Choice *A* focuses only on the liver, which is a small part of the process and not the focus of the paragraph. Choice *B* is off-track because the passage does not mention healthy foods. Choice *D* only focuses on one part of the digestive system.

54. D: The main point of this passage is to define osteoporosis. Choice *A* is incorrect because the passage does not list ways that people contract osteoporosis. Choice *B* is incorrect because the passage does not mention any treatment options. While the passage does briefly mention prevention, it does not explain how, so Choice *C* is incorrect.

55. D: The passage compares Disney cruises with Disney parks. It does not discuss how to book a cruise, so Choice *A* is incorrect. Choice *B* is incorrect because though the passage does mention some of the park attractions, it is not the main point. The passage does not mention the cost of either option, so Choice *C* is incorrect.

Vocabulary

Identifying Roots

By analyzing and understanding Latin, Greek, and Anglo-Saxon word roots and structure, authors better convey the thoughts they want to express to the readers of their words and help them to determine their meanings within the flow and without their missing a beat. For instance, **context**—how words are used in sentences—is from the Latin for *contextus*, which means "together" + "to weave," and gives readers a graphic for the minds' eyes to see the coming together of their usage. Like every other topic discussed herein, context is needed for understanding. This element actually has a second, crucial meaning. Context is not only the *how*, but the revealed moment of the *why* a writing has been composed; it is the "Aha" moment.

The way *how* words are used in sentences is important because it also gives meaning and cohesion from sentence to sentence, paragraph to paragraph, and page after page. In other words, it gives the document continuity.

Another upside of the how side is that readers have opportunities to understand new words with which they are unfamiliar. Of course, people can always look words up if a dictionary or thesaurus if available, but meaning might be gleaned on the spot in a piece that is well-written. **Synonyms** (words or phrases that mean about the same) and **antonyms** (words or phrases that mean the opposite of the specific word) in context give clues to meanings, and sometimes reiteration of a word might add clarification. Repetition, wisely used, can also serve as a part of how a piece flows.

The revealed moment of the *why* is important because context, up to that moment, has determined the shape of the text. This is, essentially, to bring out what it is all about.

Prefixes

A **prefix** is a word, letter, or number that is placed before another. It adjusts or qualifies the original word's meaning.

Four prefixes represent 97 percent of English words with prefixes. They are:

- *dis-* means "not" or "opposite of"; *dis*abled
- *in-, im-, il-, ir-* mean "not"; *il*literate
- *re-* means "again"; *re*turn
- *un-* means "not"; *un*predictable

Other commons prefixes include:

- *anti-* means "against"; *anti*bacterial
- *fore-* means "before"; *fore*front
- *mis-* means "wrongly"; *mis*understand
- *non-* means "not"; *non*sense
- *over-* means "over"; *over*abundance
- *pre-* means "before"; *pre*heat
- *super-* means "above"; *super*man

Suffixes

The official definition of a **suffix** is "a morpheme added at the end of a word to form a derivative." In English, that means a suffix is a letter or group of letters added at the end of a word to form another word. The word created with the addition is either a different tense of the same word (*help + ed = helped*) or a new word (*help + ful = helpful*).

They are:

- *-ed* is used to make present tense verbs into past tense verbs; wash*ed*
- *-ing* is used to make a present tense verb into a present participle verb; wash*ing*
- *-ly* is used to make characteristic of; love*ly*
- *-s* or *-es* are used to make more than one; chair*s* or box*es*

Other common suffixes include:

- *-able* means can be done; deplor*eable*
- *-al* means having characteristics of; comic*al*
- *-est* means comparative; great*est*
- *-ful* means full of; wonder*ful*
- *-ism* means belief in; commun*eism*
- *-less* means without; faith*less*
- *-ment* means action or process; accomplish*ment*
- *-ness* means state of; happ*yiness*
- *-ize* means to render, to make; terror*ize,* steril*ize*
- *-ise* means ditto, only this is primarily the British variant of *-ize;* surpr*ise,* advert*ise*
- -ced means go; spelling variations include -cede (concede, recede); -ceed (only three: proceed, exceed, succeed); -sede (the only one: supersede)

(Note: In some of the examples above, the *e* has been deleted.)

Word Origins

The study of the origin of a particular word, as well as how its meaning has changed over time, is called **etymology.** As an example, one might research the word *cool* and learn when *cool* became *cool* as in meanings other than in relation to *cold.*

Here are some common terms both in general usage as well as some common in medical usage:

Absence: commonly occurs in children unnoticed, is where the patient briefly loses consciousness, sometimes staring off into space, unresponsive.

Anorexia Nervosa: decreased appetite along with signs of lack of proper nutrition

Antispasmodic: a drug that has a side effect leading to excessive thirst

Arterial: referring to ulcers found in the toe area, on pressure points, and in wound that aren't healing.

Arteries: carry oxygen-rich blood away from the heart

Atonic: where the patient loses muscle tone completely throughout the body.

Attractive: having an appearance or feature that is appealing in some way.

Bereavement: can appear as a variety of different physical and other conditions such as chest pain, depression, etc.

Cerebro-vascular Accident or stroke: which a part of the brain's blood flow is restricted to a part of the brain resulting in serious, long-term or even life-threatening symptoms.

Clonic: seizure that involves the same jerking movements throughout the body.

Coma: a state of sleep in which the patient cannot be awakened either by verbal or painful stimuli.

Costly: expensive; costing a lot

Delirium: a condition involving agitation and confusion that causes a patient to lose focus and attention.

Diabetic coma: is when the blood sugar becomes so high or so low that the patient loses consciousness.

Diabetic ketoacidosis: an acidotic metabolic state in the body, resulting in an increased need to urinate, called polyuria, and excessive thirst, called polydipsia, as well as nausea, abdominal pain, fruity-scented breath, and confusion.

Displacement: a defense mechanism in which negative emotions are expressed at the wrong object.

Entire: whole; all of something

Gastroesophageal reflux or acid reflux: a common cause of chest pain that can be mistaken with a heart attack.

Gigantic: very large

Grand Mal: a seizure causing the patient to go into a state of muscle rigidity, convulsions, and unconsciousness.

Hematemesis: blood in vomit

Hematochezia: rectal bleeding

Hematopoiesis: creation of new blood cells

Hemoptysis (coughing up blood): causes include bronchitis, tuberculosis, and necrotizing pneumonia among others.

Hyperglycemia: a blood sugar of greater than 200mg/dL caused by the patient not having adequate insulin and/or anti-diabetic medication management, ingesting more glucose than normal, illness that changes normal routine, or a personal crisis that has occurred causing emotional stress in the body.

Hypoglycemia: when the blood sugar of a patient drops below 60mg/dL. Patients may develop this if they have had too much insulin or have not ingested enough dietary glucose.

Instructor: one who teaches or practices teaching

Intellectualization: a defense mechanism in which the patient focuses on thinking about their situation rather than acknowledging the associated emotions.

Isokinetic: strength exercise involving use of a machine

Isometric: strength exercise using resistance without joint motion

Isotonic: strength exercise involving joint motion

Meningitis: infection that can put a patient in a state of coma

Migraine: may cause nausea and vomiting as a side effect of their intense headache.

Myocardial infarction: or heart attack: describe chest pain as crushing and severe, with possible radiation of pain to the left arm. Their chest pain may be accompanied by sweating, nausea, shortness of breath, or a sudden weakness.

Myoclonic: causes one part of the body to make jerking movements.

Neuropathic: referring to ulcers found in feet or toe areas

Observed: to have watched to see what would happen

Pleuritis: the pleura, or lining of the lungs and chest become inflamed. This will cause a sharp sensation upon breathing, coughing, or sneezing.

Plyometrics: strength exercise combining stretching swiftly followed by contracting

Pneumonia: infection of the respiratory system that affects the lungs, may also cause the same type of sharp chest pain as pleuritic, though sometimes it may present as a deeper ache of the chest. Pneumonia will be accompanied by other signs of infection, such as fever, chills, and cough.

Reaction Formation: a defense mechanism where a person flips the emotions and act as if they are completely happy and satisfied with everything that is going on around them, often excessively so.

Residence: where one resides or lives; usually referred to as home

Seizure: characterized in a few different ways, including convulsions, disturbances in the sensory system, and even loss of consciousness.

Selecting: choosing between a number of options.

Somnolent: very sleepy, can be awakened, but will return to sleep if left alone.

Staging: refers to ulcers depending on size, tunneling as well as other factors.

Stupor: will awaken from sleep only upon painful stimuli but then return to sleep after the stimulus has discontinued.

Tonic: seizures that are characterized by a rigidity and overall stiffness of the muscles throughout the body.

Undoing: a defense mechanism in which a person does something that they regret, and then try to "undo" the action with the opposite action.

Veins: carry deoxygenated blood back to the heart.

Venous: referring to a type of ulcer found in the lower leg area

Practice Questions

1. What word meaning "on the opposite side" best fits in the following sentence? Although the patient's right knee had been hurting for a few months, he started experiencing _____ hip pain two weeks ago.
    a. Bilateral
    b. Ipsilateral
    c. Contralateral
    d. Alateral

2. Select the correct meaning of the underlined word in the following sentence. The patient's stomach appeared <u>distended</u>.
    a. Enlarged or expanded
    b. Sunken or concave
    c. Soft and flaccid
    d. Discolored or blotchy

3. What word meaning "rapidly or abruptly" best fits in the following sentence? When the school group arrived, the noise level in the waiting room rose _____.
    a. Concisely
    b. Precipitously
    c. Contingently
    d. Preemptively

4. What word meaning "open" best fits in the following sentence? After the obstruction was removed, the patient's bowel was _____.
    a. Patent
    b. Potent
    c. Evident
    d. Exude

5. What is the best definition of the word *amenorrhea*?
    a. Excessive bleeding
    b. Mental confusion
    c. Loss of appetite
    d. Absence of menstruation

6. Select the correct meaning of the underlined word in the following sentence. After the trauma, new symptoms of the woman's <u>latent</u> infection emerged.
    a. Chronic and debilitating
    b. Acute but not necessarily severe
    c. Present but not active or visible
    d. Uncontrollable or volatile

7. What word meaning "obvious" best fits in the following sentence? The patient's allergic reaction was _____, due to the widespread hives all over her extremities.
   a. Obsolete
   b. Covert
   c. Overt
   d. Colluded

8. Select the correct meaning of the underlined word in the following sentence. The nurse reported that the patient experienced <u>dyspnea</u> and dizziness.
   a. Difficulty breathing
   b. Difficulty sleeping
   c. Rapid pulse
   d. Nasal discharge

9. Select the correct meaning of the underlined word in the following sentence. The nurse explained the symptoms of the patient's <u>acute</u> illness and recommended increasing fluid intake.

   a. Serious with a poor prognosis
   b. Sudden or rapid onset
   c. Debilitating and contagious
   d. Chronic and slow to resolve

10. What word meaning "severe and harmful" best fits in the following sentence? The patient was quarantined because the doctor was concerned he had a _____ disease.
   a. Patent
   b. Innocuous
   c. Latent
   d. Virulent

11. What is the best definition of the word *adverse*?
   a. Unpredictable
   b. Agitated
   c. Undesirable
   d. Progressive

12. What word meaning "so gradual that it's hardly apparent" best fits in the following sentence? The nurse explained that atherosclerosis and coronary artery disease often have an _____ onset.
   a. Precipitous
   b. Insidious
   c. Incipient
   d. Paroxysmal

13. Select the correct meaning of the underlined word in the following sentence. The graduate student noted that the common symptoms of the condition were malaise, weight loss, and <u>anuria</u>.
   a. Lack of urine output
   b. Excessive urine production
   c. Memory loss
   d. Lack of usual reflexes

14. What word meaning "closer to the trunk" best fits in the following sentence? The knee is _____ to the ankle.
  a. Dorsal
  b. Distal
  c. Proximal
  d. Ventral

15. What word meaning "impenetrable" best fits in the following sentence? Due to the contagious nature of the patient's infection, the nursing staff was told to don _____ masks and gloves.
  a. Impotent
  b. Hygienic
  c. Impervious
  d. Impending

16. Select the correct meaning of the underlined word in the following sentence. The etiology of the disease is currently unknown.
  a. Prognosis or outlook
  b. Origin or cause
  c. Mechanism of transmission
  d. Incidence in the population

17. What word meaning "produced in the body" best fits in the following sentence? Endorphins are touted as acting as _____ opioids, to help reduce pain.
  a. Receptors
  b. Synthetic
  c. Exogenous
  d. Endogenous

18. What word meaning "feverish" best fits in the following sentence? The _____ baby was difficult to sooth.
  a. Febrile
  b. Futile
  c. Libel
  d. Liable

19. What is the best definition of the word *proliferated*?
  a. Multiplied or increased in number
  b. Responded to treatment
  c. Dwindled or decreased
  d. Expanded or grown in size

20. Select the correct meaning of the underlined word in the following sentence. The viscosity of the patient's synovial fluid was abnormal.
  a. A fluid's cellular and nutrient profile
  b. A fluid's thickness or resistance to flow
  c. A fluid's color and transparency
  d. A fluid's sedimentation rate

21. What word meaning "on one's back" best fits in the following sentence? The surgeon informed the patient that he would be _____ during the procedure.
   a. Prone
   b. Supine
   c. Dorsal
   d. Ventral

22. What is the best definition of the word *milieu*?
   a. Cytoplasm
   b. Organism
   c. Environment
   d. Autoclave

23. Select the correct meaning of the underlined word in the following sentence. The prognosis was undetermined because of the aberrant nature of his illness.
   a. Overt
   b. Grave
   c. Radical
   d. Abnormal

24. What word meaning "wound with irregular borders" best fits in the following sentence? The rock climber got a serious _____ on his arm when the boulder moved.
   a. Incision
   b. Laceration
   c. Contusion
   d. Avulsion

25. Select the correct meaning of the underlined word in the following sentence. The patient's father had a history of chronic renal disease.
   a. Relating to the pancreas
   b. Relating to the liver
   c. Relating to the kidney
   d. Relating to hormones

26. Which word meaning "removal of necrotic tissue" best fits in the following sentence? The biker was hopeful that after his knee _____, he would be in less pain.
   a. Debridement
   b. Arthroscopy
   c. Distension
   d. Laparoscopy

27. Select the correct meaning of the underlined word in the following sentence. During her internship at the hospital, Cassandra got to triage a lot of patients.
   a. Diagnose or identify a problem
   b. Develop an effective treatment plan
   c. Evaluate and gather relevant medical history
   d. Sort based on problem severity

28. What word meaning "susceptible to" best fits in the following sentence? The malnourished child was _____ to rickets.
   a. Impended
   b. Invariable
   c. Prognosticated
   d. Predisposed

29. What word meaning "to widen or expand" best fits in the following sentence? The nitrous oxide was administered to _____ his blood vessels.
   a. Dilute
   b. Dilate
   c. Occlude
   d. Distill

30. Select the correct meaning of the underlined word in the following sentence. The nurse noted that the baby appeared indolent.
   a. Underweight
   b. Agitated
   c. Lethargic
   d. Alert

31. What word referring to "blood vessels that carry deoxygenated blood back to the heart" best fits in the following sentence? The nurse was concerned about possible occlusions in the patient's _____.
   a. Capillaries
   b. Arteries
   c. Ventricles
   d. Veins

32. Select the correct meaning of the underlined word in the following sentence. The medication had a buccal route of administration.
   a. Under the tongue
   b. In the rectum
   c. Through the nasal cavity
   d. Inside the cheek

33. What is the best definition of the word *instructor*?
   a. Pupil
   b. Teacher
   c. Survivor
   d. Dictator

34. What is the best definition of the word *expectorate*?
   a. To cough out phlegm
   b. To suppress a phlegm production
   c. To stifle a cough
   d. Yellowish or green sputum

35. What is the best definition of the word *residence*?
    a. Home
    b. Area
    c. Plan
    d. Resist

36. What is the best definition of the word *relinquish*?
    a. Stop repeatedly
    b. Give again
    c. Punish again
    d. Cease claim

37. What is the best definition of the word *germinate*?
    a. Lengthen
    b. Infect
    c. Develop
    d. Ail

38. What is the best definition of the word *indemnity?*
    a. Insurance
    b. Punishment
    c. Affinity
    d. Insolation

39. Select the correct meaning of the underlined word in the following sentence. Immediately after the holiday, staff interest grew rampant.
    a. Stagnant
    b. Mildly
    c. Unrestrained
    d. Wearily

40. Select the correct meaning of the underlined word in the following sentence. An increased pupil size is considered an ominous sign.
    a. Unequivocal
    b. Promising
    c. Auspicious
    d. Threatening

41. What word meaning "low blood sugar" best fits in the following sentence? A patient with diabetes did not receive breakfast so the nurse was concerned he might have _____.
    a. Hypoglycemia
    b. Ketoacidosis
    c. Diabetic coma
    d. Hyperglycemia

42. What is the best definition of the word *observed*?
    a. Watched
    b. Hunted
    c. Scared
    d. Sold

43. What word meaning "sleepy yet arousable to verbal stimuli" best fits in the following sentence? The _____ patient was difficult to move to into the room.
    a. Comatose
    b. Delirious
    c. Somnolent
    d. Stuporous

44. What word meaning "coughing up blood" best fits in the following sentence? A patient with tuberculosis should be monitored for _____.
    a. Hematopoiesis
    b. Hemoptysis
    c. Hematemesis
    d. Hematochezia

45. What is the best definition of the word *engorge*?
    a. Nourish
    b. Squeeze
    c. Consume
    d. Swell

46. What word meaning "mourning after loss" best fits in the following sentence. The nurse referred the mother to _____ counseling.
    a. Bereavement
    b. Disposition
    c. Depression
    d. Belligerent

47. What word meaning "excessive thirst" best fits in the following sentence? A common side effect of antispasmodics is _____.
    a. Anurea
    b. Polyploidy
    c. Polydipsia
    d. Polyurea

48. What is the best definition of the word *sentient*?
    a. Kind and genial
    b. Aging or dying
    c. Able to feel or perceive
    d. Nostalgic

49. Select the correct meaning of the underlined word in the following sentence. The patient had a history of anxiety, emphysema, and a peptic ulcer.
    a. Relating to ingestion
    b. Relating to defecation
    c. Relating to digestion
    d. Relating to the pancreas

50. What word meaning "a muscle contraction that does not cause a change in muscle length" best fits in the following sentence? The strength training protocol called for many _____ exercises.

    a. Isometric
    b. Isotonic
    c. Isokinetic
    d. Plyometric

Answers

1. C: Contralateral. As a prefix, *contra-* means opposite or against. In this case, *contralateral* means on the opposite side of the body.

2. A: Enlarged or expanded. A *distended* stomach or other organ is bloated or swollen because of internal pressure.

3. B: Precipitously. *Concisely* means in a few words or efficiently worded, *contingently* refers to something that will occur only if something else happens first, and *preemptively* means something taken as a precaution or measure against an anticipated risk or problem, often as a way to try and prevent it.

4. A: Patent. In a medical context, a *patent* vessel is unobstructed and open. An atherosclerotic vessel with deposited plaques would probably not be *patent.*

5. D: Absence of menstruation. The prefix *a-* means "not" or "anti." *Menses* is the menstrual cycle, and the suffix *-rhea* means "flow." Therefore, *amenorrhea* is the absence of a menstrual period.

6. C: Present but not active or visible. A *latent* disease is present but not detectable in a symptomatic way. It may be dormant, but has to potential to become symptomatic in the future with discernable manifestations for the patient.

7. C: Overt. *Obsolete* means outdated or no longer produced or used, *covert* means not outwardly acknowledged or shown, and to *collude* is to conspire.

8. A: Difficulty breathing. The prefix *dys-* means dysfunctional or abnormal. *-Pnea* in a medical context refers to respiration and breathing. Sleep apnea is a breathing disorder that can occur during sleep.

9. B: Sudden or rapid onset. An *acute* illness is the opposite of a *chronic* one, which is a disease that the patient has had for a long time. A sinus infection is an acute illness, while multiple sclerosis is a chronic one.

10. D: Virulent. *Patent* means open, *innocuous* means harmless, and *latent* means dormant.

11. C: Undesirable. An adverse reaction to a medication is an undesirable side effect or consequence of taking the drug.

12. B: Insidious. *Precipitous* means rapid or steep, *incipient* means emergent or at an initial state, and *paroxysmal* means a sudden intensification or recurrence of symptoms, as in a paroxysmal attack of a muscle spasm in the lumbar spine.

13. A: Lack of urine output. Again, the prefixes *a-* or *an-* mean "without" or "not," and *-uria* refers to urine.

14. C: Proximal. *Distal* is the opposite of proximal. Distal means further from the trunk (usually down an extremity).

15. C: Impervious. *Impotent,* in the medical context, means unable to achieve sexual arousal (for a man). In general, the word means powerless. *Hygienic* means sanitary. *Impending* means imminent.

16. B: Origin or cause. Some diseases have an unknown etiology.

17. D: Endogenous. The prefix *endo-* means "within" or "containing," and *-genous* means originating in or producing. The prefix *exo-* means the "outside."

18. A: Febrile. *Futile* means pointless, *libel* is printed defamation of someone's character, and *liable* means responsible, especially in a legal sense.

19. A: Multiplied or increased in number. Given the right conditions, bacterial cells *proliferate* rapidly.

20. B: A fluid's thickness or resistance to flow. A viscous fluid is in contrast to a runny one. For example, honey is more viscous than water.

21. B: Supine. *Prone* is the position on one's stomach.

22. C: Environment. For example, the internal *milieu* usually refers to interstitial fluid.

23. D: Abnormal. *Overt* means outwardly demonstrative, *grave* means severe or serious, and *radical* means revolutionary or progressive.

24. B: Laceration. An *incision* is a more precise cut, as in one made by a surgeon using a scalpel during surgery. A *contusion* is a bruise and an *avulsion* is a type of fracture where a piece of the bone is ripped off.

25. C: Relating to the kidney. The renal blood vessels serve the kidneys.

26. A: Debridement. An *arthroscopy* is a type of surgical procedure on a joint using a camera and small scope, *distension* is swelling or bloating, and a *laparoscopy* is a surgical procedure that involves the insertion of a fiberoptic instrument.

27. D: Sort based on problem severity. Patients entering the ER need to be triaged so that they are treated in order of urgency.

28. D: Predisposed. *Predisposed* means inclined to a specific condition or action.

29. B: Dilate. To *dilute* is to make a solution less concentrated, *occlude* means to block or obstruct, and *distill* means to purify a liquid or to extract the most important aspects or meaning of something.

30. C: Lethargic. *Indolent* can also mean lazy or aversive to activity.

31. D: Veins. Arteries bring blood from the heart to the tissues and veins return the blood to the heart from the tissues.

32. D: Inside the cheek. An example of a medication with a buccal route of administration is nitroglycerine in the treatment of angina.

33. B: Teacher. *Pupil* means student.

34. A: To cough out phlegm. Someone with pneumonia may *expectorate* in the sink.

35. A: Home. Like the word *reside,* which means to inhabit, a *residence* is where someone lives.

36. D: To *relinquish* something is to give up claim to it. For example, a spouse trying to be more considerate may relinquish the TV remote so that his or her partner can choose a show.

37. C: To *germinate* is to develop or come into existence. A novel marketing idea might germinate at a business lunch. In a botany context, it also means to sprout or bud.

38. A: Insurance. *Indemnity* is an insurance or other security or safeguard against a financial burden or loss.

39. C: Unrestrained. *Stagnant* means still or unchanging, like a body of water with no active flow.

40. D: Threatening. Choices *B* and *C, promising* and *auspicious,* are antonyms of *ominous.*

41. A: Hypoglycemia. *Hypo-* means "below" or "beneath," and *glycemia* comes from glucose, so it refers to blood sugar.

42. A: Watched. To *observe* is to watch or examine with one's eyes.

43. C: Somnolent. Someone *comatose* is unresponsive to stimuli. Someone *delirious* is either ecstatic or mentally disturbed and seeing illusions.

44. B: Hemoptysis. The suffix *-ptysis* means spitting of matter.

45. D: Swell. A tissue that is *engorged* is swollen with fluid. For example, a new mom will have breasts engorged with milk to nurture her baby.

46. A: Bereavement. *Disposition* is someone's personality or affect, *depression* is a state of a low mood, and *belligerent* means aggressive and hostile.

47. C: Polydipsia. *Poly-* means "many" or "multiple" and the suffix *-dipsia* refers to thrist.

48. C: Able to feel or perceive. A *sentient* being is living and able to perceive or feel something and respond.

49. C: Relating to digestion. *Peptic* comes from *pepsin,* which is a stomach enzyme that helps degrade proteins.

50. A: Isometric. The prefix *iso-* means "same" and *-metric* refers to length.

Grammar

Why is grammar important? Why should we study, teach, and use proper grammar? The English language, a uniquely human achievement, deserves our consideration and examination. Language is arguably the most important tool we have for creating an impact on the world around us. Without proper grammar, language loses its efficacy for communicating well with others. Reading, writing, listening, and speaking all have a greater effect when grammar is used proficiently.

Let's begin with the basic conventions, or the **eight parts of speech***:* nouns, adjectives, adverbs, pronouns, prepositions, interjections, verbs, and conjunctions.

Parts of Speech

Nouns

A **common noun** is a word that identifies any of a class of people, places, or things. Examples include numbers, objects, animals, feelings, concepts, qualities, and actions. *A, an,* or *the* usually precedes the common noun. These parts of speech are called *articles*. Here are some examples of sentences using nouns preceded by articles.

> *A* building is under construction.

> *The* girl would like to move to *the* city.

An **abstract noun** is an idea, state, or quality. It is something that can't be touched, such as happiness, courage, evil, or humor.

A **proper noun** (also called a **proper name**) is used for the specific name of an individual person, place, or organization. The first letter in a proper noun is capitalized. "My name is *Mary*." "I work for *Walmart*."

Nouns sometimes serve as adjectives (which themselves describe nouns), such as "hockey player" and "state government."

Pronouns

A word used in place of a noun is known as a **pronoun**. Pronouns are words like *I, mine, hers,* and *us*.

Pronouns can be split into different classifications (as shown below) which make them easier to learn; however, it's not important to memorize the classifications.

- **Personal pronouns:** refer to people

- **First person pronouns:** we, I, our, mine

- **Second person pronouns:** you, yours

- **Third person pronouns:** he, them

- **Possessive pronouns:** demonstrate ownership (mine, my, his, yours)

- **Interrogative pronouns:** ask questions (what, which, who, whom, whose)

- **Relative pronouns:** include the five interrogative pronouns and others that are relative (whoever, whomever, that, when, where)

- **Demonstrative pronouns:** replace something specific (this, that, those, these)

- **Reciprocal pronouns:** indicate something was done or given in return (each other, one another)

- **Indefinite pronouns:** have a nonspecific status (anybody, whoever, someone, everybody, somebody)

Indefinite pronouns such as *anybody, whoever, someone, everybody*, and *somebody* command a singular verb form, but others such as *all, none,* and *some* could require a singular or plural verb form.

<u>Antecedents</u>
An **antecedent** is the noun to which a pronoun refers; it needs to be written or spoken before the pronoun is used. For many pronouns, antecedents are imperative for clarity. In particular, a lot of the personal, possessive, and demonstrative pronouns need antecedents. Otherwise, it would be unclear who or what someone is referring to when they use a pronoun like *he* or *this*.

Pronoun reference means that the pronoun should refer clearly to one, clear, unmistakable noun (the antecedent).

Pronoun-antecedent agreement refers to the need for the antecedent and the corresponding pronoun to agree in gender, person, and number. Here are some examples:

> The *kidneys* (plural antecedent) are part of the urinary system. *They* (plural pronoun) serve several roles."

> The kidneys are part of the *urinary system* (singular antecedent). *It* (singular pronoun) is also known as the renal system.

<u>Pronoun Cases</u>
The **subjective pronouns** —*I, you, he/she/it, we, they,* and *who*—are the subjects of the sentence.

> Example: *They* have a new house.

The **objective pronouns**—*me, you* (*singular*), *him/her, us, them,* and *whom*—are used when something is being done for or given to someone; they are objects of the action.

> Example: The teacher has an apple for *us*.

The **possessive pronouns**—*mine, my, your, yours, his, hers, its, their, theirs, our,* and *ours*—are used to denote that something (or someone) belongs to someone (or something).

> Example: It's *their* chocolate cake.

> Even Better Example: It's *my* chocolate cake!

One of the greatest challenges and worst abuses of pronouns concerns *who* and *whom*. Just knowing the following rule can eliminate confusion. *Who* is a subjective-case pronoun used only as a subject or subject complement. *Whom* is only objective-case and, therefore, the object of the verb or preposition.

> *Who* is going to the concert?

> You are going to the concert with *whom*?

Hint: When using *who* or *whom*, think of whether someone would say *he* or *him*. If the answer is *he*, use *who*. If the answer is *him*, use *whom*. This trick is easy to remember because *he* and *who* both end in vowels, and *him* and *whom* both end in the letter *M*.

Many possessive pronouns sound like contractions. For example, many people get *it's* and *its* confused. The word *it's* is the contraction for *it is*. The word *its* without an apostrophe is the possessive form of *it*.

> I love that wooden desk. It's beautiful. (contraction)

> I love that wooden desk. Its glossy finish is beautiful. (possessive)

If you are not sure which version to use, replace *it's/its* with *it is* and see if that sounds correct. If so, use the contraction (*it's*). That trick also works for *who's/whose*, *you're/your*, and *they're/their*.

Adjectives

"The *extraordinary* brain is the *main* organ of the central nervous system." The adjective *extraordinary* describes the brain in a way that causes one to realize it is more exceptional than some of other organs while the adjective *main* defines the brain's importance in its system.

An **adjective** is a word or phrase that names an attribute that describes or clarifies a noun or pronoun. This helps the reader visualize and understand the characteristics—size, shape, age, color, origin, etc.— of a person, place, or thing that otherwise might not be known. Adjectives breathe life, color, and depth into the subjects they define. Life would be *drab* and *colorless* without adjectives!

Adjectives often precede the nouns they describe.

> S*he drove her <u>new</u> car.*

However, adjectives can also come later in the sentence.

> *Her car is <u>new</u>.*

Adjectives using the prefix *a–* can only be used after a verb.

> Correct: The dog was alive until the car ran up on the curb and hit him.

> Incorrect: The alive dog was hit by a car that ran up on the curb.

Other examples of this rule include *awake, ablaze, ajar, alike,* and *asleep.*

Other adjectives used after verbs concern states of health.

> The girl was finally *well* after a long bout of pneumonia.

> The boy was *fine* after the accident.

An adjective phrase is not a bunch of adjectives strung together, but a group of words that describes a noun or pronoun and, thus, functions as an adjective. *Very ugly* is an adjective phrase; so are *way too fat* and *faster than a speeding bullet.*

Possessives

In grammar, *possessive nouns* show ownership, which was seen in previous examples like *mine, yours,* and *theirs.*

Singular nouns are generally made possessive with an apostrophe and an s ('s).

> My *uncle's* new car is silver.

> The *dog's* bowl is empty.

> *James's* ties are becoming outdated.

Plural nouns ending in *s* are generally made possessive by just adding an apostrophe ('):

> The pistachio nuts' saltiness is added during roasting. (The saltiness of pistachio nuts is added during roasting.)

> The students' achievement tests are difficult. (The achievement tests of the students are difficult.)

If the plural noun does not end in an *s* such as *women,* then it is made possessive by adding an *apostrophe s* ('s)—*women's.*

Indefinite possessive pronouns such as *nobody* or *someone* become possessive by adding an *apostrophe s*— *nobody's* or *someone's.*

Verbs

The **verb** is the part of speech that describes an action, state of being, or occurrence.

A verb forms the main part of a predicate of a sentence. This means that the verb explains what the noun (which will be discussed shortly) is doing. A simple example is *time flies*. The verb *flies* explains what the action of the noun, *time,* is doing. This example is a *main* verb.

Helping (auxiliary) verbs are words like *have, do, be, can, may, should, must,* and *will.* "I *should* go to the store." Helping verbs assist main verbs in expressing tense, ability, possibility, permission, or obligation.

Particles are minor function words like *not, in, out, up,* or *down* that become part of the verb itself. "I might *not.*"

Participles are words formed from verbs that are often used to modify a noun, noun phrase, verb, or verb phrase.

> The *running* teenager collided with the cyclist.

Participles can also create compound verb forms.

> He is *speaking*.

Participial phrases are made up of the participle and modifiers, complements, or objects.

> *Crying for most of an hour*, the baby didn't seem to want to nap.

> *Having already taken this course*, the student was bored during class.

Verbs have five basic forms: the **base** form, the **-s** form, the **-ing** form, the **past** form, and the **past participle** form.

The past forms are either **regular** (*love/loved; hate/hated*) or **irregular** because they don't end by adding the common past tense suffix "-ed" (*go/went; fall/fell; set/set*).

Adverbs

Adverbs have more functions than adjectives because they modify or qualify verbs, adjectives, or other adverbs as well as word groups that express a relation of place, time, circumstance, or cause. Therefore, adverbs answer any of the following questions: *How, when, where, why, in what way, how often, how much, in what condition,* and/or *to what degree. How good looking is he? He is <u>very</u> handsome.*

Here are some examples of adverbs for different situations:

- how: quickly
- when: daily
- where: there
- in what way: easily
- how often: often
- how much: much
- in what condition: badly
- what degree: hardly

As one can see, for some reason, many adverbs end in *-ly.*

Adverbs do things like emphasize (*really, simply,* and *so*), amplify (*heartily, completely,* and *positively*), and tone down (*almost, somewhat,* and *mildly*).

Adverbs also come in phrases.

> The dog ran as <u>though his life depended on it.</u>

Prepositions

Prepositions are connecting words and, while there are only about 150 of them, they are used more often than any other individual groups of words. They describe relationships between other words. They are placed before a noun or pronoun, forming a phrase that modifies another word in the sentence. **Prepositional phrases** begin with a preposition and end with a noun or pronoun, the **object of the preposition.** *A pristine lake is <u>near the store</u> and <u>behind the bank</u>.*

Some commonly used prepositions are *about, after, anti, around, as, at, behind, beside, by, for, from, in, into, of, off, on, to,* and *with.*

Complex prepositions, which also come before a noun or pronoun, consist of two or three words such as *according to, in regards to,* and *because of.*

Interjections

Interjections are words used to express emotion. Examples include *wow, ouch,* and *hooray.* Interjections are often separate from sentences; in those cases, the interjection is directly followed by an exclamation point. In other cases, the interjection is included in a sentence and followed by a comma. The punctuation plays a big role in the intensity of the emotion that the interjection is expressing. Using a comma or semicolon indicates less excitement than using an exclamation mark.

Conjunctions

Conjunctions are vital words that connect words, phrases, thoughts, and ideas. Conjunctions show relationships between components. There are two types:

Coordinating conjunctions are the primary class of conjunctions placed between words, phrases, clauses, and sentences that are of equal grammatical rank; the coordinating conjunctions are for, and, nor, but, or, yes, and so. A useful memorization trick is to remember that all the first letters of these conjunctions collectively spell the word fanboys.

> I need to go shopping, *but* I must be careful to leave enough money in the bank.

> She wore a black, red, *and* white shirt.

Subordinating conjunctions are the secondary class of conjunctions. They connect two unequal parts, one **main** (or **independent**) and the other **subordinate** (or **dependent**). I must go to the store *even though* I do not have enough money in the bank.

> *Because* I read the review, I do not want to go to the movie.

Notice that the presence of subordinating conjunctions makes clauses dependent. *I read the review* is an independent clause, but *because* makes the clause dependent. Thus, it needs an independent clause to complete the sentence.

Sentences

First, let's review the basic elements of sentences.

A **sentence** is a set of words that make up a grammatical unit. The words must have certain elements and be spoken or written in a specific order to constitute a complete sentence that makes sense.

> 1. A sentence must have a **subject** (a noun or noun phrase). The subject tells whom or what the sentence is addressing (i.e. what it is about).

2. A sentence must have an **action** or **state of being** (*a* verb). To reiterate: A verb forms the main part of the predicate of a sentence. This means that it explains what the noun is doing.

3. A sentence must convey a complete thought.

When examining writing, be mindful of grammar, structure, spelling, and patterns. Sentences can come in varying sizes and shapes; so, the point of grammatical correctness is not to stamp out creativity or diversity in writing. Rather, grammatical correctness ensures that writing will be enjoyable and clear. One of the most common methods for catching errors is to mouth the words as you read them. Many typos are fixed automatically by our brain, but mouthing the words often circumvents this instinct and helps one read what's actually on the page. Often, grammar errors are caught not by memorization of grammar rules but by the training of one's mind to know whether something *sounds* right or not.

Types of Sentences

There isn't an overabundance of absolutes in grammar, but here is one: every sentence in the English language falls into one of four categories.

- Declarative: a simple statement that ends with a period

    The price of milk per gallon is the same as the price of gasoline.

- Imperative: a command, instruction, or request that ends with a period

    Buy milk when you stop to fill up your car with gas.

- Interrogative: a question that ends with a question mark

    Will you buy the milk?

- Exclamatory: a statement or command that expresses emotions like anger, urgency, or surprise and ends with an exclamation mark

    Buy the milk now!

Declarative sentences are the most common type, probably because they are comprised of the most general content, without any of the bells and whistles that the other three types contain. They are, simply, declarations or statements of any degree of seriousness, importance, or information.

Imperative sentences often seem to be missing a subject. The subject is there, though; it is just not visible or audible because it is *implied*. Look at the imperative example sentence.

    Buy the milk when you fill up your car with gas.

You is the implied subject, the one to whom the command is issued. This is sometimes called *the understood you* because it is understood that *you* is the subject of the sentence.

Interrogative sentences—those that ask questions—are defined as such from the idea of the word *interrogation*, the action of questions being asked of suspects by investigators. Although that is serious business, interrogative sentences apply to all kinds of questions.

To exclaim is at the root of **exclamatory sentences**. These are made with strong emotions behind them. The only technical difference between a declarative or imperative sentence and an exclamatory one is the exclamation mark at the end. The example declarative and imperative sentences can both become an exclamatory one simply by putting an exclamation mark at the end of the sentences.

> The price of milk per gallon is the same as the price of gasoline!
> Buy milk when you stop to fill up your car with gas!

After all, someone might be really excited by the price of gas or milk, or they could be mad at the person that will be buying the milk! However, as stated before, exclamation marks in abundance defeat their own purpose! After a while, they begin to cause fatigue! When used only for their intended purpose, they can have their expected and desired effect.

Independent and Dependent Clauses

Independent and dependent clauses are strings of words that contain both a subject and a verb. An **independent clause** *can* stand alone as complete thought, but a **dependent clause** *cannot*. A dependent clause relies on other words to be a complete sentence.

> Independent clause: The keys are on the counter.
> Dependent clause: If the keys are on the counter

Notice that both clauses have a subject (*keys*) and a verb (*are*). The independent clause expresses a complete thought, but the word *if* at the beginning of the dependent clause makes it *dependent* on other words to be a complete thought.

> Independent clause: If the keys are on the counter, please give them to me.

This presents a complete sentence since it includes at least one verb and one subject and is a complete thought. In this case, the independent clause has two subjects (*keys* & an implied *you*) and two verbs (*are* & *give*).

> Independent clause: I went to the store.
> Dependent clause: Because we are out of milk,
>
> Complete Sentence: Because we are out of milk, I went to the store.
> Complete Sentence: I went to the store because we are out of milk.

Sentence Structures

A **simple sentence** has one independent clause.

> I am going to win.

A **compound sentence** has two independent clauses. A conjunction—*for, and, nor, but, or, yet, so*—links them together. Note that each of the independent clauses has a subject and a verb.

> I am going to win, but the odds are against me.

A **complex sentence** has one independent clause and one or more dependent clauses.

> I am going to win, even though I don't deserve it.

Even though I don't deserve it is a dependent clause. It does not stand on its own. Some conjunctions that link an independent and a dependent clause are *although*, *because*, *before*, *after*, *that*, *when*, *which*, and *while*.

A **compound-complex sentence** has at least three clauses, two of which are independent and at least one that is a dependent clause.

> While trying to dance, I tripped over my partner's feet, but I regained my balance quickly.

The dependent clause is *While trying to dance*.

Run-Ons and Fragments

Run-Ons

A common mistake in writing is the run-on sentence. A **run-on** is created when two or more independent clauses are joined without the use of a conjunction, a semicolon, a colon, or a dash. We don't want to use commas where periods belong. Here is an example of a run-on sentence:

> Making wedding cakes can take many hours I am very impatient, I want to see them completed right away.

There are a variety of ways to correct a run-on sentence. The method you choose will depend on the context of the sentence and how it fits with neighboring sentences:

> Making wedding cakes can take many hours. I am very impatient. I want to see them completed right away. (Use periods to create more than one sentence.)

> Making wedding cakes can take many hours; I am very impatient—I want to see them completed right away. (Correct the sentence using a semicolon, colon, or dash.)

> Making wedding cakes can take many hours, and I am very impatient and want to see them completed right away. (Correct the sentence using coordinating conjunctions.)

> I am very impatient because I would rather see completed wedding cakes right away than wait for it to take many hours. (Correct the sentence by revising.)

Fragments

Remember that a complete sentence must have both a subject and a verb. Complete sentences consist of at least one independent clause. Incomplete sentences are called **sentence fragments**. A sentence fragment is a common error in writing. Sentence fragments can be independent clauses that start with subordinating words, such as *but, as, so that,* or *because,* or they could simply be missing a subject or verb.

You can correct a fragment error by adding the fragment to a nearby sentence or by adding or removing words to make it an independent clause. For example:

> Dogs are my favorite animals. Because cats are too lazy. (Incorrect; the word because creates a sentence fragment)

> Dogs are my favorite animals because cats are too lazy. (Correct; this is a dependent clause.)

> Dogs are my favorite animals. Cats are too lazy. (Correct; this is a simple sentence.)

117

Subject and Predicate

Every complete sentence can be divided into two parts: the subject and the predicate.

Subjects: We need to have subjects in our sentences to tell us who or what the sentence describes. Subjects can be simple or complete, and they can be direct or indirect. There can also be compound subjects.

Simple subjects are the noun or nouns the sentence describes, without modifiers. The simple subject can come before or after the verb in the sentence:

> The big brown <u>dog</u> is the calmest one.

Complete subjects are the subject together with all of its describing words or modifiers.

> The <u>big brown dog</u> is the calmest one. (The complete subject is big brown dog.)

Direct subjects are subjects that appear in the text of the sentence, as in the example above. **Indirect subjects** are implied. The subject is "you," but the word *you* does not appear.

Indirect subjects usually in imperative sentences that issue a command or order:

> Feed the short skinny dog first. (The understood you is the subject.)

> Watch out—he's really hungry! (The sentence warns you to watch out.)

Compound subjects occur when two or more nouns join together to form a plural subject.

> <u>Carson</u> and <u>Emily</u> make a great couple.

Predicates: Once we have identified the subject of the sentence, the rest of the sentence becomes the predicate. Predicates are formed by the verb, the direct object, and all words related to it.

> We <u>went to see the Cirque du' Soleil performance</u>.

> The gigantic green character <u>was funnier than all the rest</u>.

A **predicate nominative** renames the subject:

> John is a <u>carpenter</u>.

A **predicate adjective** describes the subject:

> Margaret is <u>beautiful</u>.

Direct objects are the nouns in the sentence that are receiving the action. Sentences don't necessarily need objects. Sentences only need a subject and a verb.

> The clown brought the acrobat the <u>hula-hoop</u>. (What is getting brought? the hula-hoop)

> Then he gave the trick pony a <u>soapy bath</u>. (What is being given? a soapy bath)

Indirect objects are words that tell us to or for whom or what the action is being done. For there to be an indirect object, there first must always be a direct object.

> The clown brought <u>the acrobat</u> the hula-hoop. (Who is getting the direct object? the hula-hoop)

> Then he gave <u>the trick pony</u> a soapy bath. (What is getting the bath? a trick pony)

Phrases

A **phrase** is a group of words that go together but do not include both a subject and a verb. We use them to add information, explain something, or make the sentence easier for the reader to understand. Unlike clauses, phrases can never stand alone as their own sentence. They do not form complete thoughts. There are noun phrases, prepositional phrases, verbal phrases, appositive phrases, and absolute phrases. Here some examples of phrases:

> I know <u>all the shortest routes</u>.

> <u>Before the sequel</u>, we wanted to watch the first movie. (introductory phrase)

> The jumpers have hot cocoa <u>to drink right away</u>.

Subject-Verb Agreement

The subject of a sentence and its verb must agree. The cornerstone rule of subject-verb agreement is that subject and verb must agree in number. Whether the subject is singular or plural, the verb must follow suit.

> Incorrect: The houses is new.

> Correct: The houses are new.

> Also Correct: The house is new.

In other words, a singular subject requires a singular verb; a plural subject requires a plural verb.

The words or phrases that come between the subject and verb do not alter this rule.

> Incorrect: The houses built of brick is new.

> Correct: The houses built of brick are new.

> Incorrect: The houses with the sturdy porches is new.

> Correct: The houses with the sturdy porches are new.

The subject will always follow the verb when a sentence begins with *here* or *there.* Identify these with care.

> Incorrect: Here *is* the *houses* with sturdy porches.

> Correct: Here *are* the *houses* with sturdy porches.

The subject in the sentences above is not *here*, it is *houses*. Remember, *here* and *there* are never subjects. Be careful that contractions such as *here's* or *there're* do not cause confusion!

Two subjects joined by *and* require a plural verb form, except when the two combine to make one thing:

> Incorrect: Garrett and Jonathan is over there.

> Correct: Garrett and Jonathan are over there.

> Incorrect: Spaghetti and meatballs are a delicious meal!

> Correct: Spaghetti and meatballs is a delicious meal!

In the example above, *spaghetti and meatballs* is a compound noun. However, *Garrett and Jonathan* is not a compound noun.

Two singular subjects joined by *or, either/or,* or *neither/nor* call for a singular verb form.

> Incorrect: Butter or syrup are acceptable.

> Correct: Butter or syrup is acceptable.

Plural subjects joined by *or, either/or,* or *neither/nor* are, indeed, plural.

The chairs or the boxes are being moved next.

If one subject is singular and the other is plural, the verb should agree with the closest noun.

> Correct: The chair or the boxes are being moved next.

> Correct: The chairs or the box is being moved next.

Some plurals of money, distance, and time call for a singular verb.

> Incorrect: Three dollars *are* enough to buy that.

> Correct: Three dollars *is* enough to buy that.

For words declaring degrees of quantity such as *many of, some of,* or *most of,* let the noun that follows *of* be the guide:

> Incorrect: Many of the books is in the shelf.

> Correct: Many of the books are in the shelf.

> Incorrect: Most of the pie *are* on the table.

> Correct: Most of the pie *is* on the table.

For indefinite pronouns like anybody or everybody, use singular verbs.

> Everybody *is* going to the store.

However, the pronouns *few, many, several, all, some,* and *both* have their own rules and use plural forms.

> Some *are* ready.

Some nouns like *crowd* and *congress* are called *collective nouns* and they require a singular verb form.

> Congress *is* in session.

> The news *is* over.

Books and movie titles, though, including plural nouns such as *Great Expectations,* also require a singular verb. Remember that only the subject affects the verb. While writing tricky subject-verb arrangements, say them aloud. Listen to them. Once the rules have been learned, one's ear will become sensitive to them, making it easier to pick out what's right and what's wrong.

Dangling and Misplaced Modifiers

A **modifier** is a word or phrase meant to describe or clarify another word in the sentence. When a sentence has a modifier but is missing the word it describes or clarifies, it's an error called a **dangling modifier**. We can fix the sentence by revising to include the word that is being modified. Consider the following examples with the modifier underlined:

> Incorrect: <u>Having walked five miles</u>, this bench will be the place to rest. (This implies that the bench walked the miles, not the person.)

> Correct: <u>Having walked five miles</u>, Matt will rest on this bench. (*Having walked five miles* correctly modifies *Matt*, who did the walking.)

> Incorrect: <u>Since midnight</u>, my dreams have been pleasant and comforting. (The adverb clause *since midnight* cannot modify the noun *dreams*.)

> Correct: <u>Since midnight</u>, I have had pleasant and comforting dreams. (*Since midnight* modifies the verb have had, telling us when the dreams occurred.)

Sometimes the modifier is not located close enough to the word it modifies for the sentence to be clearly understood. In this case, we call the error a **misplaced modifier**. Here is an example with the modifier underlined.

> Incorrect: We gave the hot cocoa to the children <u>that was filled with marshmallows</u>. (This sentence implies that the children are what are filled with marshmallows.)

> Correct: We gave the hot cocoa <u>that was filled with marshmallows</u> to the children. (The cocoa is filled with marshmallows. The modifier is near the word it modifies.)

Parallel Structure in a Sentence

Parallel structure, also known as **parallelism**, refers to using the same grammatical form within a sentence. This is important in lists and for other components of sentences.

> Incorrect: At the recital, the boys and girls were dancing, singing, and played musical instruments.
> Correct: At the recital, the boys and girls were dancing, singing, and playing musical instruments.

Notice that in the second example, *played* is not in the same verb tense as the other verbs nor is it compatible with the helping verb *were*. To test for parallel structure in lists, try reading each item as if it were the only item in the list.

> The boys and girls were dancing.
> The boys and girls were singing.
> The boys and girls were played musical instruments.

Suddenly, the error in the sentence becomes very clear. Here's another example:

> Incorrect: After the accident, I informed the police *that Mrs. Holmes backed* into my car, *that Mrs. Holmes got out* of her car to look at the damage, and *she was driving* off without leaving a note.

> Correct: After the accident, I informed the police *that Mrs. Holmes backed* into my car, *that Mrs. Holmes got out* of her car to look at the damage, and *that Mrs. Holmes drove off* without leaving a note.

> Correct: After the accident, I informed the police that Mrs. Holmes *backed* into my car, *got out* of her car to look at the damage, and *drove off* without leaving a note.

Note that there are two ways to fix the nonparallel structure of the first sentence. The key to parallelism is consistent structure.

Punctuation

Commas

A **comma** (,) is the punctuation mark that signifies a pause—breath—between parts of a sentence. It denotes a break of flow. As with so many aspects of writing structure, authors will benefit by reading their writing aloud or mouthing the words. This can be particularly helpful if one is uncertain about whether the comma is needed.

In a complex sentence—one that contains a subordinate (dependent) clause or clauses—the use of a comma is dictated by where the subordinate clause is located. If the subordinate clause is located before the main clause, a comma is needed between the two clauses.

> I will not pay for the steak, *because I don't have that much money.*

Generally, if the subordinate clause is placed after the main clause, no punctuation is needed. I did well on my exam because I studied two hours the night before. Notice how the last clause is dependent because it requires the earlier independent clauses to make sense.

Use a comma on both sides of an interrupting phrase.

> I will pay for the ice cream, chocolate and vanilla, and then will eat it all myself.

The words forming the phrase in italics are nonessential (extra) information. To determine if a phrase is nonessential, try reading the sentence without the phrase and see if it's still coherent.

A comma is not necessary in this next sentence because no interruption—nonessential or extra information—has occurred. Read sentences aloud when uncertain.

I will pay for his chocolate and vanilla ice cream and then will eat it all myself.

If the nonessential phrase comes at the beginning of a sentence, a comma should only go at the end of the phrase. If the phrase comes at the end of a sentence, a comma should only go at the beginning of the phrase.

Other types of interruptions include the following:

- interjections: Oh no, I am not going.
- abbreviations: Barry Potter, M.D., specializes in heart disorders.
- direct addresses: Yes, Claudia, I am tired and going to bed.
- parenthetical phrases: His wife, lovely as she was, was not helpful.
- transitional phrases: Also, it is not possible.

The second comma in the following sentence is called an Oxford comma.

> I will pay for ice cream, syrup, and pop.

It is a comma used after the second-to-last item in a series of three or more items. It comes before the word *or* or *and*. Not everyone uses the Oxford comma; it is optional, but many believe it is needed. The comma functions as a tool to reduce confusion in writing. So, if omitting the Oxford comma would cause confusion, then it's best to include it.

Commas are used in math to mark the place of thousands in numerals, breaking them up so they are easier to read. Other uses for commas are in dates (*March 19, 2016*), letter greetings (*Dear Sally,*), and in between cities and states (*Louisville, KY*).

Apostrophes

This punctuation mark, the apostrophe ('), is a versatile little mark. It has a few different functions:

- Quotes: Apostrophes are used when a second quote is needed within a quote.

- In my letter to my friend, I wrote, "The girl had to get a new purse, and guess what Mary did? She said, 'I'd like to go with you to the store.' I knew Mary would buy it for her."

- Contractions: Another use for an apostrophe in the quote above is a contraction. *I'd* is used for *I would.*

The basic rule for making *contractions* is one area of spelling that is pretty straightforward: combine the two words by inserting an apostrophe (') in the space where a letter is omitted. For example, to combine *you* and *are*, drop the *a* and put the apostrophe in its place: *you're*.

> he + is = he's
>
> you + all = y'all (informal but often misspelled)

- Possession: An apostrophe followed by the letter *s* shows possession (*Mary's* purse). If the possessive word is plural, the apostrophe generally just follows the word.

- The trees' leaves are all over the ground.

Ellipses

An **ellipsis** (...) consists of three handy little dots that can speak volumes on behalf of irrelevant material. Writers use them in place of a word(s), line, phrase, list contents, or paragraph that might just as easily have been omitted from a passage of writing. This can be done to save space or to focus only on the specifically relevant material.

> Exercise is good for some unexpected reasons. Watkins writes, "Exercise has many benefits such as ...reducing cancer risk."

In the example above, the ellipsis takes the place of the other benefits of exercise that are more expected.

The ellipsis may also be used to show a pause in sentence flow.

> "I'm wondering...how this could happen," Dylan said in a soft voice.

Semicolons

The **semicolon** (;) might be described as a heavy-handed comma. Take a look at these two examples:

> I will pay for the ice cream, but I will not pay for the steak.
> I will pay for the ice cream; I will not pay for the steak.

What's the difference? The first example has a comma and a conjunction separating the two independent clauses. The second example does not have a conjunction, but there are two independent clauses in the sentence, so something more than a comma is required. In this case, a semicolon is used.

Two independent clauses can only be joined in a sentence by either a comma and conjunction or a semicolon. If one of those tools is not used, the sentence will be a run-on. Remember that while the clauses are independent, they need to be closely related in order to be contained in one sentence.

Another use for the semicolon is to separate items in a list when the items themselves require commas.

> The family lived in Phoenix, Arizona; Oklahoma City, Oklahoma; and Raleigh, North Carolina.

Colons

Colons (:) have many miscellaneous functions. Colons can be used to proceed further information or a list. In these cases, a colon should only follow an independent clause.

> Humans take in sensory information through five basic senses: sight, hearing, smell, touch, and taste.

The meal includes the following components:

- Caesar salad
- spaghetti
- garlic bread
- cake

The family got what they needed: a reliable vehicle.

While a comma is more common, a colon can also proceed a formal quotation.

> He said to the crowd: "Let's begin!"

The colon is used after the greeting in a formal letter.

> Dear Sir:
> To Whom It May Concern:

In the writing of time, the colon separates the minutes from the hour (*4:45 p.m.*). The colon can also be used to indicate a ratio between two numbers (*50:1*).

Hyphens

The **hyphen** (-) is a little hash mark that can be used to join words to show that they are linked.

Hyphenate two words that work together as a single adjective (a compound adjective).

> honey-covered biscuits

Some words always require hyphens, even if not serving as an adjective.

> merry-go-round

Hyphens always go after certain prefixes like *anti-* & *all-*.

Hyphens should also be used when the absence of the hyphen would cause a strange vowel combination (*semi-engineer*) or confusion. For example, *re-collect* should be used to describe something being gathered twice rather than being written as *recollect*, which means to remember.

Parentheses and Dashes

Parentheses are half-round brackets that look like this: ( ). They set off a word, phrase, or sentence that is a afterthought, explanation, or side note relevant to the surrounding text but not essential. A pair of commas is often used to set off this sort of information, but parentheses are generally used for information that would not fit well within a sentence or that the writer deems not important enough to be structurally part of the sentence.

> The picture of the heart (see above) shows the major parts you should memorize.
> Mount Everest is one of three mountains in the world that are over 28,000 feet high (K2 and Kanchenjunga are the other two).

See how the sentences above are complete without the parenthetical statements? In the first example, *see above* would not have fit well within the flow of the sentence. The second parenthetical statement could have been a separate sentence, but the writer deemed the information not pertinent to the topic.

The **dash** (—) is a mark longer than a hyphen used as a punctuation mark in sentences and to set apart a relevant thought. Even after plucking out the line separated by the dash marks, the sentence will be intact and make sense.

> Looking out the airplane window at the landmarks—Lake Clarke, Thompson Community College, and the bridge—she couldn't help but feel excited to be home.

The dashes use is similar to that of parentheses or a pair of commas. So, what's the difference? Many believe that using dashes makes the clause within them stand out while using parentheses is subtler. It's advised to not use dashes when commas could be used instead.

Quotation Marks

Here are some instances where *quotation marks* should be used:

- Dialogue for characters in narratives. When characters speak, the first word should always be capitalized and the punctuation goes inside the quotes. For example:

  > Janie said, "The tree fell on my car during the hurricane."

- Around titles of songs, short stories, essays, and chapter in books
- To emphasize a certain word
- To refer to a word as the word itself

Capitalization

Here's a non-exhaustive list of things that should be capitalized.

- The first word of every sentence
- The first word of every line of poetry
- The first letter of proper nouns (World War II)
- Holidays (Valentine's Day)
- The days of the week and months of the year (Tuesday, March)
- The first word, last word, and all major words in the titles of books, movies, songs, and other creative works (In the novel, *To Kill a Mockingbird*, note that *a* is lowercase since it's not a major word, but *to* is capitalized since it's the first word of the title.)
- Titles when preceding a proper noun (President Roberto Gonzales, Aunt Judy)

When simply using a word such as president or secretary, though, the word is not capitalized.

> Officers of the new business must include a *president* and *treasurer*.

Seasons—spring, fall, etc.—are not capitalized.

North, *south*, *east*, and *west* are capitalized when referring to regions but are not when being used for directions. In general, if it's preceded by *the* it should be capitalized.

> I'm from the South.
> I drove south.

Writing Tips

Conciseness

Unfortunately, writers often include extra words and phrases that seem necessary at the time but add nothing to the main idea. This confuses the reader and creates unnecessary repetition. Writing that lacks conciseness is usually guilty of excessive wordiness and redundant phrases. Here's an example containing both of these issues:

> When legislators decided to begin creating legislation making it mandatory for automobile drivers and passengers to make use of seat belts while in cars, a large number of them made those laws for reasons that were political reasons.

There are several empty or "luff words here that take up too much space. These can be eliminated while still maintaining the writer's meaning. For example:

- "Decided to begin" could be shortened to "began"
- "Making it mandatory for" could be shortened to "requiring"
- "Make use of" could be shortened to "use"
- "A large number" could be shortened to "many"

In addition, there are several examples of redundancy that can be eliminated:

- "Legislators decided to begin creating legislation" and "made those laws"
- "Automobile drivers and passengers" and "while in cars"
- "Reasons that were political reasons"

These changes are incorporated as follows:

> When legislators began requiring drivers and passengers to use seat belts, many of them did so for political reasons.

Euphemisms

Eliminating **euphemisms** can be helpful in writing more concisely. Euphemisms are terms or phrases used to say something indirectly. Often times it's to soften an expression, be polite, or in some cases to be impolite.

Normal expression: He is very short.

Euphemism: He is vertically challenged.

Clichés

A **cliché** is an old, often-used phrase that has lost all originality or humor due to it's overuse. These idioms are all *clichés*:

A penny for your thoughts

Head over heels in love

Give your two cents

It's best to avoid clichés since they are overused and because their elimination can help you be more concise.

Distinguishing Between Formal and Informal Language

It can be helpful to distinguish whether a writer or speaker is using formal or informal language because it can give the reader or listener clues to whether the text is informative, nonfiction, argumentative, or the intended tone or audience. Formal and informal language in written or verbal communication serve different purposes and are often intended for different audiences. Consequently, their tone, word choices, and grammatical structures vary. These differences can be used to identify which form of language is used in a given piece and to determine which type of language should be used for a certain context. Understanding the differences between formal and informal language will also allow a writer or speaker to implement the most appropriate and effective style for a given situation.

Formal language is less personal and more informative and pragmatic than informal language. It is more "buttoned-up" and business-like, adhering to proper grammatical rules. It is used in professional or academic contexts, to convey respect or authority. For example, one would use formal language to write an informative or argumentative essay for school and to address a superior or esteemed professional like a potential employer, a professor, or a manager. Formal language avoids contractions, slang, colloquialisms, and first-person pronouns.

Informal language is often used when communicating with family members, friends, peers, and those known more personally. It is more casual, spontaneous, and forgiving in its conformity to grammatical rules and conventions. Informal language is used for personal emails, some light fiction stories, and some correspondence between coworkers or other familial relationships.

Slang refers to non-standard expressions that are not used in elevated speech and writing. Slang creates linguistic in-groups and out-groups of people, those who can understand the slang terms and those who can't. Slang is often tied to a specific time period. For example, "groovy" and "far out" are connected to the 1970s, and "as if!" and "4-1-1-" are connected to the 1990s. **Colloquial language** is language that is used conversationally or familiarly—e.g., "What's up?"—in contrast to formal, professional, or academic language—"How are you this evening?" Formal language uses sentences that are usually more complex and often in passive voice. Punctuation can differ as well. For example, exclamation points are used to show strong emotion or can be used as an interjection but should be used sparingly in formal writing situations.

Textspeak is a term used to refer to the informal language used in text messages and similar messaging mediums. While often appropriate for use in those contexts, it should be avoided in more formal settings.

Outside of casual conversations, it's important to use formal language both in speaking and writing.

Sensitivity

In speech and writing, it's important to be cognizant as to how your words are perceived by others. Racist, sexist, and other derogatory language should be avoided because it is rude, demeaning, and can severely hurt career opportunities. It may be helpful to adopt a position of being "above reproach", meaning that your words and actions are so pure they cannot be criticized for being insensitive.

Word Confusion

That/Which
The pronouns *that* and *which* are both used to refer to animals, objects, ideas, and events—but they are not interchangeable. The rule is to use the word *that* in essential clauses and phrases that are help convey the meaning of the sentence. Use the word *which* in nonessential (less important) clauses. Typically, *which* clauses are enclosed in commas.

The morning <u>that I fell asleep in class</u> caused me a lot of trouble.

This morning's coffee, <u>which had too much creamer</u>, woke me up.

Who/Whom
We use the pronouns *who* and *whom* to refer to people. We always use *who* when it is the subject of the sentence or clause. We never use *whom* as the subject; it is always the object of a verb or preposition.

<u>Who</u> hit the baseball for the home run? (subject)

The baseball fell into the glove of <u>whom</u>? (object of the preposition of)

The umpire called <u>whom</u> "out"? (object of the verb called)

To/Too/Two
to: a preposition or infinitive (*to walk, to run, walk to the store, run to the tree*)
too: means also, as well, or very (*She likes cookies, too.; I ate too much.*)
two: a number (*I have two cookies. She walked to the store two times.*)

There/Their/They're
there: an adjective, adverb, or pronoun used to start a sentence or indicate place (*There are four vintage cars over there.*)
their: a possessive pronoun used to indicate belonging (*Their car is the blue and white one.*)
they're: a contraction of the words "they are" (*They're going to enter the vintage car show.*)

Your/You're

> your: a possessive pronoun (*Your artwork is terrific.*)
> you're: a contraction of the words "you are" (*You're a terrific artist.*)

Its/It's

> its: a possessive pronoun (*The elephant had its trunk in the water.*)
> it's: a contraction of the words "it is" (*It's an impressive animal.*)

Affect/Effect

> affect: as a verb means "to influence" (*How will the earthquake affect your home?*); as a noun means "emotion or mood" (*Her affect was somber.*)
> effect: as a verb means "to bring about" (*She will effect a change through philanthropy.*); as a noun means "a result of" (*The effect of the earthquake was devastating.*)

> Other mix-ups: Other pairs of words cause mix-ups but are not necessarily homonyms. Here are a few of those:

Bring/Take

> bring: when the action is coming toward (*Bring me the money.*)
> take: when the action is going away from (*Take her the money.*)

Can/May

> can: means "able to" (*The child can ride a bike.*)
> may: asks permission (*The child asked if he may ride his bike.*)

Than/Then

> than: a conjunction used for comparison (*I like tacos better than pizza.*)
> then: an adverb telling when something happened (*I ate and then slept.*)

Disinterested/Uninterested

> disinterested: used to mean "neutral" (*The jury remains disinterested during the trial.*)
> uninterested: used to mean "bored" (*I was uninterested during the lecture.*)

Percent/Percentage

> percent: used when there is a number involved (*Five percent of us like tacos.*)
> percentage: used when there is no number (*That is a low percentage.*)

Fewer/Less

> fewer: used for things you can count (*He has fewer playing cards.*)
> less: used for things you cannot count, as well as time (*He has less talent. You have less than a minute.*)

Farther/Further

> farther: used when discussing distance (*His paper airplane flew farther than mine.*)
> further: used to mean "more" (*He needed further information.*)

Lend/Loan

> lend: a verb used for borrowing (*Lend me your lawn mower. He will lend it to me.*)
> loan: a noun used for something borrowed (*She applied for a student loan.*)

<u>Note</u>
Some people have problems with these:

- regardless/irregardless
- a lot/alot

Irregardless and *alot* are always incorrect. Don't use them.

Please keep in mind that grammar questions on the actual exam may be hospital related.

Practice Questions

1. Which of the following sentences has an error in capitalization?
   a. The East Coast has experienced very unpredictable weather this year.
   b. My Uncle owns a home in Florida, where he lives in the winter.
   c. I am taking English Composition II on campus this fall.
   d. There are several nice beaches we can visit on our trip to the Jersey Shore this summer.

2. Julia Robinson, an avid photographer in her spare time, was able to capture stunning shots of the local wildlife on her last business trip to Australia.
Which of the following is an adjective in the preceding sentence?
   a. Time
   b. Capture
   c. Avid
   d. Photographer

3. Which of the following sentences uses correct punctuation?
   a. Carole is not currently working; her focus is on her children at the moment.
   b. Carole is not currently working and her focus is on her children at the moment.
   c. Carole is not currently working, her focus is on her children at the moment.
   d. Carole is not currently working her focus is on her children at the moment.

4. Which of these examples is a compound sentence?
   a. Alex and Shane spent the morning coloring and later took a walk down to the park.
   b. After coloring all morning, Alex and Shane spent the afternoon at the park.
   c. Alex and Shane spent the morning coloring, and then they took a walk down to the park.
   d. After coloring all morning and spending part of the day at the park, Alex and Shane took a nap.

5. Which of these examples shows incorrect use of subject-verb agreement?
   a. Neither of the cars are parked on the street.
   b. Both of my kids are going to camp this summer.
   c. Any of your friends are welcome to join us on the trip in November.
   d. Each of the clothing options is appropriate for the job interview.

6. When it gets warm in the spring, _____ and _____ like to go fishing at Cobbs Creek.
Which of the following word pairs should be used in the blanks above?
   a. me, him
   b. he, I
   c. him, I
   d. he, me

7. Which example shows correct comma usage for dates?
   a. The due date for the final paper in the course is Monday, May 16, 2016.
   b. The due date for the final paper in the course is Monday, May 16 2016.
   c. The due date for the final project in the course is Monday, May, 16, 2016.
   d. The due date for the final project in the course is Monday May 16, 2016.

8. At last night's company function, in honor of Mr. Robertson's retirement, several employees spoke kindly about his career achievements.

In the preceding sentence, what part of speech is the word *function*?
   a. Adjective
   b. Adverb
   c. Verb
   d. Noun

9. Which of the examples uses the correct plural form?
   a. Tomatos
   b. Analysis
   c. Cacti
   d. Criterion

10. Which of the following examples uses correct punctuation?
   a. The moderator asked the candidates, "Is each of you prepared to discuss your position on global warming?".
   b. The moderator asked the candidates, "Is each of you prepared to discuss your position on global warming?"
   c. The moderator asked the candidates, 'Is each of you prepared to discuss your position on global warming?'
   d. The moderator asked the candidates, "Is each of you prepared to discuss your position on global warming"?

11. In which of the following sentences does the word *part* function as an adjective?
   a. The part Brian was asked to play required many hours of research.
   b. She parts ways with the woodsman at the end of the book.
   c. The entire team played a part in the success of the project.
   d. Ronaldo is part Irish on his mother's side of the family.

12. All of Shannon's family and friends helped her to celebrate her 50th birthday at Café Sorrento. Which of the following is the complete subject of the preceding sentence?
   a. Family and friends
   b. All
   c. All of Shannon's family and friends
   d. Shannon's family and friends

13. Which of the following examples correctly uses quotation marks?
   a. "Where the Red Fern Grows" was one of my favorite novels as a child.
   b. Though he is famous for his roles in films like "The Great Gatsby" and "Titanic," Leonardo DiCaprio has never won an Oscar.
   c. Sylvia Plath's poem, "Daddy" will be the subject of this week's group discussion.
   d. "The New York Times" reported that many fans are disappointed in some of the trades made by the Yankees this off-season.

14. Which of the following sentences shows correct word usage?
    a. It's often been said that work is better then rest.
    b. Its often been said that work is better then rest.
    c. It's often been said that work is better than rest.
    d. Its often been said that work is better than rest.

15. Which of the following is an imperative sentence?
    a. Pennsylvania's state flag includes two draft horses and an eagle.
    b. Go down to the basement and check the hot water heater for signs of a leak.
    c. You must be so excited to have a new baby on the way!
    d. How many countries speak Spanish?

16. Which of the following examples is a compound sentence?
    a. Shawn and Jerome played soccer in the backyard for two hours.
    b. Marissa last saw Elena and talked to her this morning.
    c. The baby was sick, so I decided to stay home from work.
    d. Denise, Kurt, and Eric went for a run after dinner.

17. Which of the following sentences uses correct subject-verb agreement?
    a. There is two constellations that can be seen from the back of the house.
    b. At least four of the sheep needs to be sheared before the end of summer.
    c. Lots of people were auditioning for the singing competition on Saturday.
    d. Everyone in the group have completed the assignment on time.

18. Philadelphia is home to some excellent walking tours where visitors can learn more about the culture and rich history of the city of brotherly love.
What are the adjectives in the preceding sentence?
    a. Philadelphia, tours, visitors, culture, history, city, love
    b. Excellent, walking, rich, brotherly
    c. Is, can, learn
    d. To, about, of

19. The realtor showed _____ and _____ a house on Wednesday afternoon.
Which of the following pronoun pairs should be used in the blanks above?
    a. She, I
    b. She, me
    c. Me, her
    d. Her, me

20. Which of the following examples uses correct punctuation?
    a. Recommended supplies for the hunting trip include the following: rain gear, large backpack, hiking boots, flashlight, and non-perishable foods.
    b. I left the store, because I forgot my wallet.
    c. As soon as the team checked into the hotel; they met in the lobby for a group photo.
    d. None of the furniture came in on time: so they weren't able to move in to the new apartment.

21. Which of the following sentences shows correct word usage?
    a. Your going to have to put you're jacket over their.
    b. You're going to have to put your jacket over there.
    c. Your going to have to put you're jacket over they're.
    d. You're going to have to put your jacket over their.

22. A teacher notices that, when students are talking to each other between classes, they are using their own unique vocabulary words and expressions to talk about their daily lives. When the teacher hears these non-standard words that are specific to one age or cultural group, what type of language is she listening to?
    a. Slang
    b. Jargon
    c. Dialect
    d. Vernacular

23. A teacher wants to counsel a student about using the word *ain't* in a research paper for a high school English class. What advice should the teacher give?
    a. *Ain't* is not in the dictionary, so it isn't a word.
    b. Because the student isn't in college yet, *ain't* is an appropriate expression for a high school writer.
    c. *Ain't* is incorrect English and should not be part of a serious student's vocabulary because it sounds uneducated.
    d. *Ain't* is a colloquial expression, and while it may be appropriate in a conversational setting, it is not standard in academic writing.

24. What is the structure of the following sentence?
    The restaurant is unconventional because it serves both Chicago style pizza and New York style pizza.

    a. Simple
    b. Compound
    c. Complex
    d. Compound-complex

25. The following sentence contains what kind of error?
    This summer, I'm planning to travel to Italy, take a Mediterranean cruise, going to Pompeii, and eat a lot of Italian food.

    a. Parallelism
    b. Sentence fragment
    c. Misplaced modifier
    d. Subject-verb agreement

26. The following sentence contains what kind of error?
    Forgetting that he was supposed to meet his girlfriend for dinner, Anita was mad when Fred showed up late.

    a. Parallelism
    b. Run-on sentence
    c. Misplaced modifier
    d. Subject-verb agreement

27. The following sentence contains what kind of error?
    Some workers use all their sick leave, other workers cash out their leave.

    a. Parallelism
    b. Comma splice
    c. Sentence fragment
    d. Subject-verb agreement

28. A student writes the following in an essay:
    Protestors filled the streets of the city. Because they were dissatisfied with the government's leadership.

Which of the following is an appropriately-punctuated correction for this sentence?
    a. Protestors filled the streets of the city, because they were dissatisfied with the government's leadership.
    b. Protesters, filled the streets of the city, because they were dissatisfied with the government's leadership.
    c. Because they were dissatisfied with the government's leadership protestors filled the streets of the city.
    d. Protestors filled the streets of the city because they were dissatisfied with the government's leadership.

29. What is the part of speech of the underlined word in the sentence?
    We need to come up with a fresh <u>approach</u> to this problem.

    a. Noun
    b. Verb
    c. Adverb
    d. Adjective

30. What is the part of speech of the underlined word in the sentence?
    Investigators conducted an <u>exhaustive</u> inquiry into the accusations of corruption.

    a. Noun
    b. Verb
    c. Adverb
    d. Adjective

31. The underlined portion of the sentence is an example of which sentence component?
    New students should report <u>to the student center</u>.

    a. Dependent clause
    b. Adverbial phrase
    c. Adjective clause
    d. Noun phrase

32. Which word choices will correctly complete the sentence?

Increasing the price of bus fares has had a greater [affect / effect] on ridership [then / than] expected.

a. affect; then
b. affect; than
c. effect; then
d. effect; than

33. The following is an example of what type of sentence?

Although I wished it were summer, I accepted the change of seasons, and I started to appreciate the fall.

a. Compound
b. Simple
c. Complex
d. Compound-Complex

34. A student reads the following sentence:

A hundred years ago, automobiles were rare, but now cars are ubiquitous.

However, she doesn't know what the word *ubiquitous* means. Which key context clue is essential to decipher the word's meaning?

a. Ago
b. Cars
c. Now
d. Rare

35. Which word in the following sentence is a proper noun?

People think the Statue of Liberty is an awesome sight.
a. People
b. Statue of Liberty
c. Awesome
d. Sight

36. Which word in the following sentence is a plural noun?

The black kitten was the girl's choice from the litter of kittens.
a. Kitten
b. Girl's
c. Choice
d. Kittens

37. Which pronoun makes the following sentence grammatically correct?

_____ ordered the flowers?
a. Whose
b. Whom
c. Who
d. Who've

38. Which pronoun makes the following sentence grammatically correct?

    The giraffe nudged _____ baby.
    a. it's
    b. hers
    c. their
    d. its

39. What is the word *several* in the following sentence called?

    Several are laughing loudly on the bus.
    a. Singular indefinite pronoun
    b. Plural indefinite pronoun
    c. Singular objective pronoun
    d. Indefinite adjective

40. Which word in the following sentence is an adjective?

    The connoisseur slowly enjoyed the delectable meal.
    a. Delectable
    b. Connoisseur
    c. Slowly
    d. Enjoyed

41. Which choice identifies all of the prepositions in the following sentence?

    We went down by the water, near the lake, before dawn, to see the pretty sunrise.
    a. Went, to see, pretty
    b. By, near, before
    c. Water, lake, dawn, sunrise
    d. We, down, the, pretty

42. Which sentence has an interjection?
    a. The cookie was full of chocolaty goodness.
    b. Well, Carrie didn't like the cookie.
    c. Can't you see that cookie is broken?
    d. That's too bad, but I'll still eat it!

43. Identify the complete subject in the following sentence.

    The heaviest green bike is mine.
    a. bike
    b. green bike
    c. The heaviest green bike
    d. is mine

44. Identify the complete predicate in the following sentence.

    My house is the yellow one at the end of the street.
    a. My house
    b. is the yellow one
    c. at the end of the street.
    d. is the yellow one at the end of the street.

45. Which sentence shows incorrect subject/verb agreement?
    a. All of the kittens in the litter show their courage.
    b. The black kitten pounce on the ball of yarn.
    c. The calico kitten eats voraciously.
    d. My favorite kitten snuggles with its mother.

46. What is the indirect object in the following sentence?
    Calysta brought her mother the beautiful stained-glass lamp.
    a. Stained-glass lamp
    b. Brought
    c. Her mother
    d. Beautiful

47. Which sentence is grammatically correct?
    a. They're on their way to New Jersey but there not there yet.
    b. Their on their way to New Jersey but they're not there yet.
    c. They're on their way to New Jersey but they're not there yet.
    d. They're on their way to New Jersey but there not their yet.

48. Identify the prepositional phrase in the following sentence.
    For the longest time, I have wanted to learn to roller skate.
    a. I have wanted
    b. wanted to learn
    c. learn to roller skate
    d. For the longest time

49. Identify the sentence structure of the following sentence.
    The weight of the world was on his shoulders, so he took a long walk.
    a. Simple sentence
    b. Compound sentence
    c. Complex sentence
    d. Compound-complex sentence

50. Identify the sentence structure of the following sentence.
    The last thing she wanted to do was see the Eiffel Tower before the flight.
    a. Simple sentence
    b. Compound sentence
    c. Complex sentence
    d. Compound-complex sentence

51. Which of the following sentences is a fragment?
    a. We went to the zoo to see the tigers and lions.
    b. Instead we saw elephants, zebras and giraffes.
    c. Because the lion and tiger habitat was closed.
    d. What sound does a giraffe make anyway?

52. Which of the following is a run-on sentence?
    a. I love to go water-skiing, I love alpine skiing, I also love Nordic skiing.
    b. The best way to learn to ski is to take lessons.
    c. All three types of skiing require different skills and different equipment.
    d. It takes a long time to learn how to ski; waterskiing takes the longest time.

53. Which sentence has a dangling modifier?
    a. Eating a large meal, I had to chew my food slowly.
    b. Eating a large meal, my food had to be chewed slowly.
    c. Eating a large meal, I was too full afterward.
    d. Eating a large meal, I was more full than I have ever been.

54. Which sentence has a misplaced modifier?
    a. The children love their cute and cuddly teddy bears.
    b. Teddy bears are cute and cuddly; the children love them.
    c. Cute and cuddly, the children love their teddy bears.
    d. Cute and cuddly, the teddy bears are loved by many children.

55. Which sentence shows grammatically correct parallelism?
    a. The puppies enjoy chewing and to play tug-o-war.
    b. The puppies enjoy to chew and playing tug-o-war.
    c. The puppies enjoy to chew and to play tug-o-war.
    d. The puppies enjoy chewing and playing tug-o-war.

Answer Explanations

1. B: In choice B the word *Uncle* should not be capitalized, because it is not functioning as a proper noun. If the word named a specific uncle, such as *Uncle Jerry*, then it would be considered a proper noun and should be capitalized. Choice *A* correctly capitalizes the proper noun *East Coast*, and does not capitalize *winter*, which functions as a common noun in the sentence. Choice *C* correctly capitalizes the name of a specific college course, which is considered a proper noun. Choice *D* correctly capitalizes the proper noun *Jersey Shore*.

2. C: In choice C, *avid* is functioning as an adjective that modifies the word photographer. *Avid* describes the photographer Julia Robinson's style. The words *time* and *photographer* are functioning as nouns, and the word *capture* is functioning as a verb in the sentence. Other words functioning as adjectives in the sentence include, *local*, *business*, and *spare*, as they all describe the nouns they precede.

3. A: Choice *A* is correctly punctuated because it uses a semicolon to join two independent clauses that are related in meaning. Each of these clauses could function as an independent sentence. Choice *B* is incorrect because the conjunction is not preceded by a comma. A comma and conjunction should be used together to join independent clauses. Choice *C* is incorrect because a comma should only be used to join independent sentences when it also includes a coordinating conjunction such as *and* or *so*. Choice *D* does not use punctuation to join the independent clauses, so it is considered a fused (same as a run-on) sentence.

4. C: Choice *C* is a compound sentence because it joins two independent clauses with a comma and the coordinating conjunction *and*. The sentences in Choices B and D include one independent clause and one dependent clause, so they are complex sentences, not compound sentences. The sentence in Choice *A* has both a compound subject, *Alex and Shane*, and a compound verb, *spent and took*, but the entire sentence itself is one independent clause.

5. A: Choice *A* uses incorrect subject-verb agreement because the indefinite pronoun *neither* is singular and must use the singular verb form *is*. The pronoun *both* is plural and uses the plural verb form of *are*. The pronoun *any* can be either singular or plural. In this example, it is used as a plural, so the plural verb form *are* is used. The pronoun *each* is singular and uses the singular verb form *is*.

6. B: Choice *B* is correct because the pronouns *he* and *I* are in the subjective case. *He* and *I* are the subjects of the verb *like* in the independent clause of the sentence. Choice A, C, and D are incorrect because they all contain at least one objective pronoun (*me* and *him*). Objective pronouns should not be used as the subject of the sentence, but rather, they should come as an object of a verb. To test for correct pronoun usage, try reading the pronouns as if they were the only pronoun in the sentence. For example, *he* and *me* may appear to be the correct answer choices, but try reading them as the only pronoun.

> He like[s] to go fishing...

> Me like to go fishing...

> When looked at that way, *me* is an obviously incorrect choice.

7. A: It is necessary to put a comma between the date and the year. It is also required to put a comma between the day of the week and the month. Choice *B* is incorrect because it is missing the comma between the day and year. Choice *C* is incorrect because it adds an unnecessary comma between the month and date. Choice *D* is missing the necessary comma between day of the week and the month.

8. D: In Choice D, the word function is a noun. While the word *function* can also act as a verb, in this particular sentence it is acting as a noun as the object of the preposition *at*. Choices A and B are incorrect because the word *function* cannot be used as an adjective or adverb.

9. C: Cacti is the correct plural form of the word *cactus*. Choice A (*tomatos*) includes an incorrect spelling of the plural of *tomato*. Both choice B (*analysis*) and choice D (*criterion*) are incorrect because they are in singular form. The correct plural form for these choices would be *criteria* and analyses.

10. B: Quotation marks are used to indicate something someone said. The example sentences feature a direct quotation that requires the use of double quotation marks. Also, the end punctuation, in this case a question mark, should always be contained within the quotation marks. Choice A is incorrect because there is an unnecessary period after the quotation mark. Choice C is incorrect because it uses single quotation marks, which are used for a quote within a quote. Choice D is incorrect because it places the punctuation outside of the quotation marks.

11. D: In choice D, the word *part* functions as an adjective that modifies the word *Irish*. Choices A and C are incorrect because the word *part* functions as a noun in these sentences. Choice B is incorrect because the word *part* functions as a verb.

12. C: *All of Shannon's family and friends* is the complete subject because it includes who or what is doing the action in the sentence as well as the modifiers that go with it. Choice *A* is incorrect because it only includes the simple subject of the sentence. Choices B and D are incorrect because they only include part of the complete subject.

13. C: Choice *C* is correct because quotation marks should be used for the title of a short work such as a poem. Choices A, B, and D are incorrect because the titles of novels, films, and newspapers should be placed in italics, not quotation marks.

14. C: This question focuses on the correct usage of the commonly confused word pairs of *it's/its* and *then/than*. *It's* is a contraction for *it is* or *it has*. *Its* is a possessive pronoun. The word *than* shows comparison between two things. *Then* is an adverb that conveys time. Choice C correctly uses *it's* and *than*. *It's* is a contraction for *it has* in this sentence, and *than* shows comparison between *work* and *rest*. None of the other answers choices use both of the correct words.

15. B: Choice *B* is an imperative sentence because it issues a command. In addition, it ends with a period, and an imperative sentence must end in a period or exclamation mark. Choice A is a declarative sentence that states a fact and ends with a period. Choice C is an exclamatory sentence that shows strong emotion and ends with an exclamation point. Choice D is an interrogative sentence that asks a question and ends with a question mark.

16. C: Choice *C* is a compound sentence because it joins two independent clauses—*The baby was sick* and *I decided to stay home from work*—with a comma and the coordinating conjunction *so*. Choices A, B, and D, are all simple sentences, each containing one independent clause with a complete subject and predicate. Choices A and D each contain a compound subject, or more than one subject, but they are still simple sentences that only contain one independent clause. Choice *B* contains a compound verb (more than one verb), but it's still a simple sentence.

17. C: The simple subject of this sentence, the word *lots*, is plural. It agrees with the plural verb form *were*. Choice *A* is incorrect, because the simple subject *there*, referring to the two constellations, is considered plural. It does not agree with the singular verb form *is*. In Choice *B*, the plural subject *four*, does not agree with the singular verb form *needs*. In Choice *D* the singular subject *everyone* does not agree with the third person plural verb form *have*.

18. B: *Excellent* and *walking* are adjectives modifying the noun *tours*. *Rich* is an adjective modifying the noun *history*, and *brotherly* is an adjective modifying the noun *love*. Choice *A* is incorrect because all of these words are functioning as nouns in the sentence. Choice *C* is incorrect because all of these words are functioning as verbs in the sentence. Choice *D* is incorrect because all of these words are considered prepositions, not adjectives.

19. D: The object pronouns *her* and *me* act as the indirect objects of the sentence. If *me* is in a series of object pronouns, it should always come last in the series. Choice *A* is incorrect because it uses subject pronouns *she* and *I*. Choice *B* is incorrect because it uses the subject pronoun *she*. Choice *C* uses the correct object pronouns, but they are in the wrong order.

20. A: In this example, a colon is correctly used to introduce a series of items. Choice *B* places an unnecessary comma before the word *because*. A comma is not needed before the word *because* when it introduces a dependent clause at the end of a sentence and provides necessary information to understand the sentence. Choice *C* is incorrect because it uses a semi-colon instead of a comma to join a dependent clause and an independent clause. Choice *D* is incorrect because it uses a colon in place of a comma and coordinating conjunction to join two independent clauses.

21. B: Choice *B* correctly uses the contraction for *you are* as the subject of the sentence, and it correctly uses the possessive pronoun *your* to indicate ownership of the jacket. It also correctly uses the adverb *there*, indicating place. Choice *A* is incorrect because it reverses the possessive pronoun *your* and the contraction for *you are*. It also uses the possessive pronoun *their* instead of the adverb *there*. Choice *C* is incorrect because it reverses *your* and *you're* and uses the contraction for *they are* in place of the adverb *there*. Choice *D* incorrectly uses the possessive pronoun *their* instead of the adverb *there*.

22. A: Slang refers to non-standard expressions that are not used in elevated speech and writing. Slang tends to be specific to one group or time period and is commonly used within groups of young people during their conversations with each other. Jargon refers to the language used in a specialized field. The vernacular is the native language of a local area, and a dialect is one form of a language in a certain region. Thus, *B*, *C*, and *D* are incorrect.

23. D: Colloquial language is that which is used conversationally or informally, in contrast to professional or academic language. While *ain't* is common in conversational English, it is a non-standard expression in academic writing. For college-bound students, high school should introduce them to the expectations of a college classroom, so *B* is not the best answer. Teachers should also avoid placing moral or social value on certain patterns of speech. Rather than teaching students that their familiar speech patterns are bad, teachers should help students learn when and how to use appropriate forms of expression, so *C* is wrong. *Ain't* is in the dictionary, so *A* is incorrect, both in the reason for counseling and in the factual sense.

24. C: A complex sentence joins an independent or main clause with a dependent or subordinate clause. In this case, the main clause is "The restaurant is unconventional." This is a clause with one subject-verb combination that can stand alone as a grammatically-complete sentence. The dependent clause is "because it serves both Chicago style pizza and New York style pizza." This clause begins with the subordinating conjunction *because* and also consists of only one subject-verb combination. *A* is incorrect because a simple sentence consists of only one verb-subject combination—one independent clause. *B* is incorrect because a compound sentence contains two independent clauses connected by a conjunction. *D* is incorrect because a complex-compound sentence consists of two or more independent clauses and one or more dependent clauses.

25. A: Parallelism refers to consistent use of sentence structure or word form. In this case, the list within the sentence does not utilize parallelism; three of the verbs appear in their base form—*travel, take*, and *eat*—but one appears as a gerund—*going*. A parallel version of this sentence would be "This summer, I'm planning to travel to Italy, take a Mediterranean cruise, go to Pompeii, and eat a lot of Italian food." *B* is incorrect because this description is a complete sentence. *C* is incorrect as a misplaced modifier is a modifier that is not located appropriately in relation to the word or words they modify. *D* is incorrect because subject-verb agreement refers to the appropriate conjugation of a verb in relation to its subject.

26. C: In this sentence, the modifier is the phrase "Forgetting that he was supposed to meet his girlfriend for dinner." This phrase offers information about Fred's actions, but the noun that immediately follows it is Anita, creating some confusion about the "do-er" of the phrase. A more appropriate sentence arrangement would be "Forgetting that he was supposed to meet his girlfriend for dinner, Fred made Anita mad when he showed up late." *A* is incorrect as parallelism refers to the consistent use of sentence structure and verb tense, and this sentence is appropriately consistent. *B* is incorrect as a run-on sentence does not contain appropriate punctuation for the number of independent clauses presented, which is not true of this description. *D* is incorrect because subject-verb agreement refers to the appropriate conjugation of a verb relative to the subject, and all verbs have been properly conjugated.

27. B: A comma splice occurs when a comma is used to join two independent clauses together without the additional use of an appropriate conjunction. One way to remedy this problem is to replace the comma with a semicolon. Another solution is to add a conjunction: "Some workers use all their sick leave, but other workers cash out their leave." *A* is incorrect as parallelism refers to the consistent use of sentence structure and verb tense; all tenses and structures in this sentence are consistent. *C* is incorrect because a sentence fragment is a phrase or clause that cannot stand alone—this sentence contains two independent clauses. *D* is incorrect because subject-verb agreement refers to the proper conjugation of a verb relative to the subject, and all verbs have been properly conjugated.

28. D: The problem in the original passage is that the second sentence is a dependent clause that cannot stand alone as a sentence; it must be attached to the main clause found in the first sentence. Because the main clause comes first, it does not need to be separated by a comma. However, if the dependent clause came first, then a comma would be necessary, which is why Choice *C* is incorrect. *A* and *B* also insert unnecessary commas into the sentence.

29. A: A noun refers to a person, place, thing, or idea. Although the word *approach* can also be used as a verb, in the sentence it functions as a noun within the noun phrase "a fresh approach," so *B* is incorrect. An adverb is a word or phrase that provides additional information of the verb, but because the verb is *need* and not *approach*, then *C* is false. An adjective is a word that describes a noun, used here as the word *fresh*, but it is not the noun itself. Thus, *D* is also incorrect.

30. D: An adjective modifies a noun, answering the question "Which one?" or "What kind?" In this sentence, the word *exhaustive* is an adjective that modifies the noun *investigation*. Another clue that this word is an adjective is the suffix *–ive*, which means "having the quality of." The nouns in this sentence are *investigators, inquiry, accusations,* and *corruption*; therefore, *A* is incorrect. The verb in this sentence is *conducted* because this was the action taken by the subject *the investigators*; therefore, *B* is incorrect. *C* is incorrect because an adverb is a word or phrase that provides additional information about the verb, expressing how, when, where, or in what manner.

31. B: In this case, the phrase functions as an adverb modifying the verb *report*, so *B* is the correct answer. "To the student center" does not consist of a subject-verb combination, so it is not a clause; thus, Choices *A* and *C* can be eliminated. This group of words is a phrase. Phrases are classified by either the controlling word in the phrase or its function in the sentence. *D* is incorrect because a noun phrase is a series of words that describe or modify a noun.

32. D: In this sentence, the first answer choice requires a noun meaning *impact* or *influence*, so *effect* is the correct answer. For the second answer choice, the sentence is drawing a comparison. *Than* shows a comparative relationship whereas *then* shows sequence or consequence. *A* and *C* can be eliminated because they contain the choice *then*. *B* is incorrect because *affect* is a verb while this sentence requires a noun.

33. D: Since the sentence contains two independent clauses and a dependent clause, the sentence is categorized as compound-complex:

> Independent clause: *I accepted the change of seasons*

> Independent clause: *I started to appreciate the fall*

> Dependent clause: *Although I wished it were summer*

34. D: Students can use context clues to make a careful guess about the meaning of unfamiliar words. Although all of the words in a sentence can help contribute to the overall sentence, in this case, the adjective that pairs with *ubiquitous* gives the most important hint to the student—cars were first *rare*, but now they are *ubiquitous*. The inversion of *rare* is what gives meaning to the rest of the sentence and *ubiquitous* means "existing everywhere" or "not rare." *A* is incorrect because *ago* only indicates a time frame. *B* is incorrect because *cars* does not indicate a contrasting relationship to the word *ubiquitous* to provide a good context clue. *C* is incorrect because it also only indicates a time frame, but used together with *rare*, it provides the contrasting relationship needed to identify the meaning of the unknown word.

35. B: Proper nouns are specific. *Statue of Liberty* is a proper noun and specifies exactly which statue is being discussed. Choice *A* is incorrect because the word *people* is a common noun and it is only capitalized because it is at the beginning of the sentence. Choice *C* is incorrect. The word *awesome* is an adjective describing the sight. Choice *D* is incorrect. The word *sight* is a common noun. A clue to eliminate answer choices *C* and *D* is that they were not capitalized. Proper nouns are always capitalized.

36. D: The word *kittens* is plural, meaning more than one kitten. Choice *A* is incorrect. The word *kitten* is singular. Choice *B* is incorrect. The word *girl's* is a singular possessive form. The girl is making the choice. There is only one girl involved. Choice *C* is incorrect. The word *choice* is a singular noun. The girl has only one choice to make. The word *litter* in this sentence is a collective plural noun meaning a group of kittens.

37. C: The word *who* in the sentence is a subjective interrogative pronoun and the sentence needed a subject that begins a question. Choice *A* is incorrect. The word *whose* is a possessive pronoun and it is not being asked who owns the flowers. Choice *B* is incorrect. The word *whom* is always an objective pronoun—never a subjective one; a subjective pronoun is needed in this sentence. Choice *D* is incorrect. The word *who've* is a contraction of the words *who* and *have*. We would not say, *"Who have ordered the flowers?"*

38. D: The word *its* in the sentence is the singular possessive form of the pronoun that stands in place for the word *giraffe's.* There is one baby that belongs to one giraffe. Choice *A* is incorrect. It is a contraction of the words *it* and *is.* You would not say, *"The giraffe nudged it is baby."* Choice *B* is incorrect. We do not know the gender of the giraffe and if it was female the proper word would be *her* baby not *hers* baby. Choice *C* is incorrect. The word *their* is a plural possessive pronoun and we need a singular possessive pronoun because there is only one giraffe doing the nudging.

39. B: The word *several* stands in for a plural noun at the beginning of the sentence, such as the noun *people*. It is also an indefinite pronoun because the number of people, for example, is not defined. Choice *A* is incorrect. The pronoun is plural not singular. It indicates more than one person. We can tell because the sentence works with the plural word *are* for the verb; substituting the singular word *is* would not make sense. We wouldn't say, *"Several is laughing loudly on the bus."* Choice *C* is incorrect. *Several* is the subject of the sentence. Therefore, it is a subjective pronoun not an objective one. Choice *D* is incorrect. The word *several* does not modify a noun in the sentence. If the sentence said, *"Several people are laughing loudly on the bus,"* then the word *several* would be an indefinite adjective modifying the word *people*.

40. A: The word *delectable* is an adjective modifying the noun *meal* in the sentence. It answers the question: *"What kind of meal?"* Choice *B* is incorrect. The word *connoisseur* is a noun that is the subject of the sentence. Choice *C* is incorrect. The word *slowly* is an adverb telling how the subject enjoyed the meal. Choice *D* is incorrect. The word *enjoyed* is the past-tense verb in the sentence telling us what action the subject had taken.

41. B: The word *by* is a positional preposition telling where we are in relation to the water. The word *near* is also a positional preposition telling where *we* are in relation to the lake. The word *before* is a time preposition telling when in relation to the time of day, dawn. Choice *A* is incorrect because *went* and *to see* are both verbs and *pretty* is an adjective modifying the word *sunrise*. Choice *C* is incorrect because *water, lake, dawn,* and *sunrise* are all nouns in the sentence. Choice *D* is incorrect because the word *we* is a pronoun, the word *down* is an adverb modifying the verb *went*, the word *the* is an article, and the word *pretty* is an adjective modifying *sunrise*.

42. B: The word *well* at the beginning of the sentence is set apart from the rest of the sentence with a comma and is a mild interjection. Choice *A* is incorrect. The word *goodness* at the end of the sentence is a noun. It is the idea/state of being for the cookie. Choice *C* is incorrect. It is an interrogative sentence and all of the words in the sentence can be identified as other parts of speech. *Can't* is a contraction of the word cannot and it works with the word *see* as the verb in the sentence. The word *you* is a pronoun; the word *that* is an adjective modifying the word *cookie*; *cookie* is a noun; *is* is another verb; and *broken* is an adjective modifying the word *cookie*. Choice *D* is incorrect because the exclamation mark at the end of the sentence is not there to set apart an interjection. Rather, it is there to punctuate the exclamatory sentence.

43. C: The simple subject is *bike* and its modifiers *the heaviest* and *green* are included to form the complete subject. Choice *A* is incorrect because *bike* is the simple subject. Choice *B* is incorrect because it includes only one of the modifiers (*green*) of the word *bike*. Choice *D* is incorrect because *is mine* is the predicate of the sentence, not the subject.

44. D: The subject of the sentence is *my house;* therefore, the rest of the sentence is the predicate. Choice *A* is incorrect because *my house* is the subject, not the predicate. Choice *B* is incorrect because *is the yellow one* is only part of the predicate, but the sentence does not end there. Choice *C* is incorrect because *at the end of the street* is only a portion of the predicate.

45. B: The *kitten* is a singular subject and so the singular verb *pounces* should be used instead of *pounce*. Choice *A* is incorrect because the plural subject *kittens* agrees with the plural verb *show*. Choice *C* is incorrect because the singular subject *kitten* agrees with the singular verb *eats*. Choice *D* is incorrect because the singular subject *kitten* agrees with the singular verb *snuggles*.

46. C: *Her mother* is to whom Calysta brought the lamp. Choice *A* is incorrect because *stained-glass lamp* is the direct object of the sentence. Choice *B* is incorrect because *brought* is the verb. Choice *D* is incorrect because *beautiful* is an adjective modifying the noun *lamp*.

47. C: *They're* (they are) on *their* (possessive) way to New Jersey but *they're* (they are) not *there* (location) yet. This sentence makes sense. Choice *A* is incorrect because after the word *but* should be the word *they're* (they are). Choice *B* is incorrect because the sentence should begin with *they're* (they are) instead of *their* (possessive). Choice *D* is incorrect because after the word *not* should be *there* (location) instead of *their* (possessive).

48. D: *For the longest time* is an introductory prepositional phrase beginning with the preposition *for* and all the modifiers for the word *time*. Choice *A* is incorrect because it includes the past-tense verb *have wanted* creating a clause. Choice *B* is incorrect because it includes the verb *wanted* and the infinitive *to learn*. Choice *C* is incorrect because it includes the verb *learn* and the infinitive *to skate*.

49. B: *The weight of the world was on his shoulders* and *he took a long walk* are both independent clauses connected with a comma and a coordinating conjunction. Choice *A* is incorrect because there are two independent clauses and a simple sentence has only one independent clause. Choice *C* is incorrect because the sentence has no dependent clauses and a complex sentence needs at least one dependent clause. Choice *D* is incorrect because, although there are two independent clauses, there are no dependent clauses and a compound-complex sentence will have at least two independent clauses and at least one dependent clause.

50. A: *The last thing she wanted to do was see the Eiffel Tower before the flight* has only one independent clause and no dependent clauses therefore it is a simple sentence. Choice *B* is incorrect because the sentence has only one independent clause. *The last thing she wanted to do* is a gerund phrase serving as the noun subject of the sentence, therefore it is not an independent clause. Choice *C* is incorrect because the sentence has no dependent clauses therefore it cannot be a complex sentence. Choice *D* is incorrect because the sentence has only one independent clause and no dependent clauses. A compound-complex sentence needs at least two independent clauses and at least one dependent clause.

51. C: *Because the lion and tiger habitat was closed* is a dependent clause and needs a subject. Choice *A* is incorrect because the sentence is an independent clause with both a subject and a verb, therefore it creates a complete sentence. Choice *B* is incorrect because the sentence is also a complete independent clause. Choice *D* is incorrect because the sentence is a complete independent clause forming an interrogative sentence.

52. A: *I love to go water-skiing, I love alpine skiing,* and *I also love Nordic skiing* are all independent clauses and are not connected with coordinating conjunctions or separated with semi colons, colons, or dashes. This makes it a run-on sentence. Choice *B* is not a run-on sentence; it is a simple single independent clause. Choice *C* is incorrect; it is a complete independent clause with both a subject (*types of skiing*) and a verb (*require*). Choice *D* is incorrect. It contains two independent clauses but a semicolon correctly separates them, therefore it is a complete compound sentence.

53. B: *Eating a large meal* cannot modify the word *food*. The food is not eating the meal. Choice *A* does not contain a dangling modifier. *Eating a large meal* modifies the pronoun *I*. Choice *C* does not contain a dangling modifier. It contains an incorrect preposition. The sentence should say, "*After eating a large meal, I was too full.*" Choice *D* does not contain a dangling modifier. *Eating a large meal* correctly modifies the pronoun *I*. *I* ate the large meal.

54. C: The dependent adjective clause *cute and cuddly* does not modify *the children*, it modifies *teddy bears*. The modifier is misplaced. Choice *A* does not contain a misplaced modifier. It is a grammatically correct independent clause. Choice *B* does not have a misplaced modifier. It is a grammatically correct compound sentence with two independent clauses joined with a semicolon. Choice *D* does not have a misplaced modifier. The modifier *cute and cuddly* correctly modifies *teddy bears*. The sentence is grammatically correct.

55. D: To create parallelism, make both verbal gerunds. Choice *A* is incorrect. *Chewing* is a gerund and *to play* is an infinitive. Choice *B* is incorrect. *To chew* is an infinitive and *playing* is a gerund. Choice *C* is incorrect. *To chew* and *to play* are both infinitives, but they do not match with the verb *enjoy*.

Biology

Biology is the study of living organisms and the processes that are vital for life.

Biology Basics

Taxonomy is the science behind the biological names of organisms. Biologists often refer to organisms by their Latin scientific names to avoid confusion with common names, such as with fish. Jellyfish, crayfish, and silverfish all have the word "fish" in their name, but belong to three different species. In the eighteenth century, Carl Linnaeus invented a naming system for species that included using the Latin scientific name of a species, called the *binomial*, which has two parts: the *genus*, which comes first, and the *specific epithet*, which comes second. Similar species are grouped into the same genus. The Linnean system is the commonly used taxonomic system today and, moving from comprehensive similarities to more general similarities, classifies organisms into their species, genus, family, order, class, phylum, and kingdom. *Homo sapiens* is the Latin scientific name for humans.

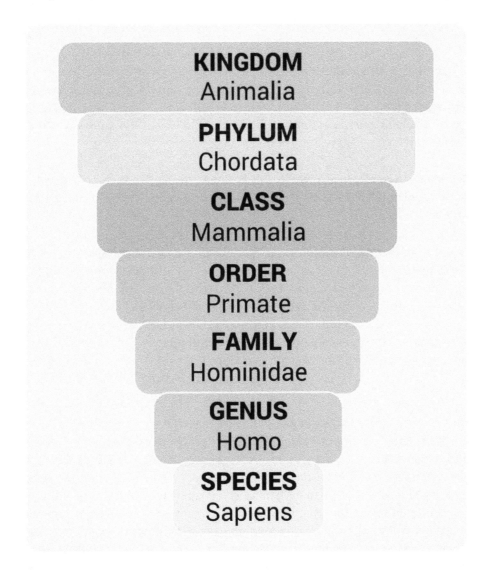

Scientific Method

Human beings are, by nature, very curious. Long before the scientific method was established, people have been making observations and predicting outcomes, manipulating the physical world to create extraordinary things—from the first man-made fire in 6000 B.C.E. to the satellite that orbited Pluto in 2016. Although the history of the scientific method is sporadic and attributed to many different people, it remains the most reliable way to obtain and utilize knowledge about the observable universe. The scientific method consists of the following steps:

- **Make an observation:** An **observation** is the analysis of information using basic human senses: sight, sound, touch, taste, and smell. Observations can be two different types—qualitative or quantitative. A *qualitative observation* describes what is being observed, such as the color of a house or the smell of a flower. *Quantitative observations* measure what is being observed, such as the number of windows on a house or the intensity of a flower's smell on a scale of 1-5.

- **Create a question:** Observations lead to the identification of a problem, also called an **inference**. Inferences are logical predictions based on experience or education that lead to the formation of a hypothesis.

- **Form a hypothesis:** A **hypothesis** is a testable explanation of an observed scenario and is presented in the form of a statement. It's an attempt to answer a question based on an observation, and it allows a scientist to predict an outcome. A hypothesis makes assumptions on the relationship between two different variables, and answers the question: "If I do this, what happens to that?"

- **Conduct an experiment:** Once a hypothesis has been formed, it must be tested to determine whether it's true or false. To test a hypothesis, one must conduct a carefully designed experiment.

- **Collect and analyze data:** Once the experiment begins, a disciplined scientist must always record the observations in meticulous detail, usually in a journal. Upon reading this journal, a different scientist should be able to clearly understand the experiment and recreate it exactly. The journal includes all **collected data**, or any observed changes.

- **Form a conclusion:** The final step of the scientific method is to make inferences from observed data, which is also known as forming a **conclusion**.

Water

Most cells are primarily composed of water and live in water-rich environments. Since water is such a familiar substance, it is easy to overlook its unique properties. Chemically, water is made up of two hydrogen atoms bonded to one oxygen atom by covalent bonds. The three atoms join to make a V-shaped molecule. Water is a polar molecule, meaning it has an unevenly distributed overall charge due to an unequal sharing of electrons. Due to oxygen's electronegativity and its more substantial positively charged nucleus, hydrogen's electrons are pulled closer to the oxygen. This causes the hydrogen atoms to have a slight positive charge and the oxygen atom to have a slight negative charge. In a glass of water, the molecules constantly interact and link for a fraction of a second due to intermolecular bonding between the slightly positive hydrogen atoms of one molecule and the slightly negative oxygen of a different molecule. These weak intermolecular bonds are called **hydrogen bonds**.

Water has several important qualities, including: cohesive and adhesive behaviors, temperature moderation ability, expansion upon freezing, and diverse use as a solvent.

Cohesion is the interaction of many of the same molecules. In water, cohesion occurs when there is hydrogen bonding between water molecules. Water molecules use this bonding ability to attach to each other and can work against gravity to transport dissolved nutrients to the top of a plant. A network of water-conducting cells can push water from the roots of a plant up to the leaves. Adhesion is the linking of two different substances. Water molecules can form a weak hydrogen bond with, or adhere to, plant cell walls to help fight gravity. The cohesive behavior of water also causes surface tension. If a glass of water is slightly overfull, water can still stand above the rim. This is because of the unique bonding of water molecules at the surface—they bond to each other and to the molecules below them, making it seem like it is covered with an impenetrable film. A raft spider could actually walk across a small body of water due to this surface tension.

Another important property of water is its ability to moderate temperature. Water can moderate the temperature of air by absorbing or releasing stored heat into the air. Water has the distinctive capability of being able to absorb or release large quantities of stored heat while undergoing only a small change in temperature. This is because of the relatively high **specific heat** of water, where specific heat is the amount of heat it takes for one gram of a material to change its temperature by 1 degree Celsius. The specific heat of water is one calorie per gram per degree Celsius, meaning that for each gram of water, it takes one calorie of heat to raise or lower the temperature of water by 1 degree Celsius.

When the temperature of water is reduced to freezing levels, water displays another interesting property: It expands instead of contracts. Most liquids become denser as they freeze because the molecules move around slower and stay closer together. Water molecules, however, form hydrogen bonds with each other as they move together. As the temperature lowers and they begin to move slower, these bonds become harder to break apart. When water freezes into ice, molecules are frozen with hydrogen bonds between them and they take up about 10 percent more volume than in their liquid state. The fact that ice is less dense than water is what makes ice float to the top of a glass of water.

Lastly, the **polarity** of water molecules makes it a versatile solvent. **Ionic compounds**, such as salt, are made up of positively- and negatively-charged atoms, called **cations** and **anions**, respectively. Cations and anions are easily dissolved in water because of their individual attractions to the slight positive charge of the hydrogen atoms or the slight negative charge of the oxygen atoms in water molecules. Water molecules separate the individually charged atoms and shield them from each other so they don't bond to each other again, creating a homogenous solution of the cations and anions. Nonionic compounds, such as sugar, have polar regions, so are easily dissolved in water. For these compounds, the water molecules form hydrogen bonds with the polar regions (hydroxyl groups) to create a homogenous solution. Any substance that is attracted to water is termed **hydrophilic**. Substances that repel water are termed **hydrophobic**.

Biological Molecules

Basic units of organic compounds are often called **monomers**. Repeating units of linked monomers are called **polymers**. The most important large molecules, or polymers, found in all living things can be divided into four categories: carbohydrates, lipids, proteins, and nucleic acids. This may be surprising since there is so much diversity in the outward appearance and physical abilities of living things present on Earth. Carbon (C), hydrogen (H), oxygen (O), nitrogen (N), sulfur (S), and phosphorus (P) are the major elements of most biological molecules. Carbon is a common backbone of large molecules because of its ability to form four covalent bonds.

Carbohydrates

Carbohydrates consist of sugars and polymers of sugars. The simplest sugar are **monosaccharide**, which have the empirical formula of CH_2O. The formula for the monosaccharide glucose, for example, is $C_6H_{12}O_6$. Glucose is an important molecule for cellular respiration, the process of cells extracting energy by breaking bonds through a series of reactions. The individual atoms are then used to rebuild new small molecules. **Polysaccharides** are made up of a few hundred to a few thousand monosaccharides linked together. These larger molecules have two major functions. The first is that they can be stored as starches, such as **glycogen**, and then broken down later for energy. Secondly, they may be used to form strong materials, such as **cellulose**, which is the firm wall that encloses plant cells, and **chitin**, the carbohydrate insects use to build exoskeletons.

Lipids

Lipids are a class of biological molecules that are **hydrophobic**, meaning they don't mix well with water. They are mostly made up of large chains of carbon and hydrogen atoms, termed **hydrocarbon chains**. When lipids mix with water, the water molecules bond to each other and exclude the lipids because they are unable to form bonds with the long hydrocarbon chains. Because the structure of different lipids is so diverse, they have a wide range of functions, which include energy storage, signaling, structure, protection, and making up the cell membrane. The three most important types of lipids are fats, phospholipids, and steroids.

Fats are made up of two types of smaller molecules: glycerol and fatty acids. **Glycerol** is a chain of three carbon atoms, with a **hydroxyl group** attached to each carbon atom. A hydroxyl group is made up of an oxygen and hydrogen atom bonded together. **Fatty acids** are long hydrocarbon chains that have a backbone of sixteen or eighteen carbon atoms. The carbon atom on one end of the fatty acid is part of a **carboxyl group.** A carboxyl group is a carbon atom that uses two of its four bonds to bond to one oxygen atom (double bond) and uses another one of its bonds to link to a hydroxyl group.

Fats are made by joining three fatty acid molecules and one glycerol molecule.

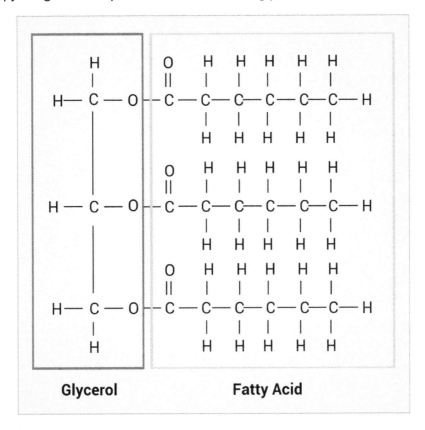

These energy-storage molecules can exist as any of the following types.

- **Saturated fats** have no double bonds within their fatty acid tails. These are solid at room temperature and are mostly animal fats like bacon fat.

- **Unsaturated fats** have double bonds within any of their fatty acid tails. Due to the kinks caused by the double bonds, these fats are liquid at room temperature and are mostly plant fats like olive oil.

Phospholipids are made of two fatty acid molecules linked to one glycerol molecule. A **phosphate group** is attached to a third hydroxyl group of the glycerol molecule. A phosphate group consists of a phosphate atom connected to four oxygen atoms and has an overall negative charge.

Phospholipids have an interesting structure because their fatty acid tails are hydrophobic, but their phosphate group heads are hydrophilic. When phospholipids mix with water, they create double-layered structures, called **bilayers,** that shield their hydrophobic regions from water molecules. Cell membranes are made of phospholipid bilayers, which allow the cells to mix with aqueous solutions outside and inside, while forming a protective barrier and a semi-permeable membrane around the cell.

Steroids are lipids that consist of four fused carbon rings. The different chemical groups that attach to these rings are what make up the many types of steroids. **Cholesterol** is a common type of steroid found in animal cell membranes. Steroids are mixed in between the phospholipid bilayer and help maintain the structure of the membrane and aids in cell signaling.

Proteins

Proteins are essential for most all functions in living beings. The term *protein* is derived from the Greek word *proteios*, meaning *first* or *primary*. All proteins are made from a set of twenty **amino acids**, molecules that are linked in unbranched polymers. The combinations are numerous, which accounts for the diversity of proteins. Amino acids are linked by peptide bonds, while polymers of amino acids are called **polypeptides**. These polypeptides, either individually or in linked combination with each other, fold up to form coils of biologically-functional molecules, called proteins.

There are four levels of protein structure: primary, secondary, tertiary, and quaternary. The **primary structure** is the sequence of amino acids, similar to the letters in a long word. The **secondary structure** is beta sheets, or alpha helices, formed by hydrogen bonding between the polar regions of the polypeptide backbone. **Tertiary structure** is the overall shape of the molecule that results from the interactions between the side chains linked to the polypeptide backbone. **Quaternary structure** is the overall protein structure that occurs when a protein is made up of two or more polypeptide chains.

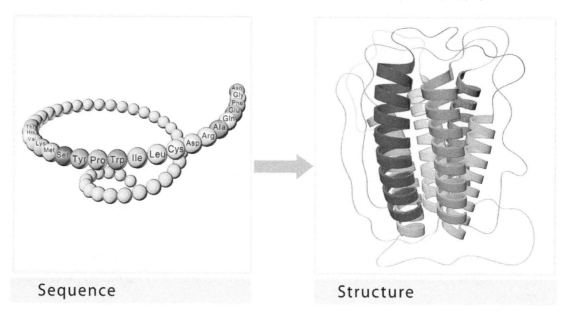

Sequence   Structure

Nucleic Acids

Nucleic acids can also be called **polynucleotides** because they are made up of chains of monomers called **nucleotides.** Nucleotides consist of a five-carbon sugar, a nitrogen-containing base, and a phosphate group. There are two types of nucleic acids: **deoxyribonucleic acid (DNA)** and **ribonucleic acid (RNA)**. Both DNA and RNA enable living organisms to pass on their genetic information and complex components to subsequent generations. While DNA is made up of two strands of nucleotides coiled together in a double-helix structure, RNA is made up of a single strand of nucleotides that folds onto itself.

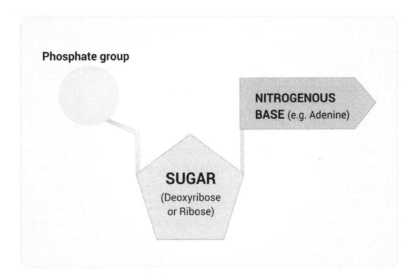

Metabolism

Metabolism is the set of chemical processes that occur within a cell for the maintenance of life. It includes both the synthesizing and breaking down of substances. A **metabolic pathway** begins with a molecule and ends with a specific product after going through a series of reactions, often involving an enzyme at each step. An **enzyme** is a protein that aids in the reaction. **Catabolic pathways** are metabolic pathways in which energy is released by complex molecules being broken down into simpler molecules. Contrast to catabolic pathways are **anabolic pathways**, which use energy to build complex molecules out of simple molecules. With cell metabolism, remember the **first law of thermodynamics**: Energy can be transformed, but it cannot be created or destroyed. Therefore, the energy released in a cell by a catabolic pathway is used up in anabolic pathways.

The reactions that occur within metabolic pathways are classified as either exergonic reactions or endergonic reactions. **Exergonic reactions** end in a release of free energy, while **endergonic reactions** absorb free energy from its surroundings. **Free energy** is the portion of energy in a system, such as a living cell, that can be used to perform work, such as a chemical reaction. It is denoted as the capital letter G and the change in free energy from a reaction or set of reactions is denoted as delta G (ΔG). When reactions do not require an input of energy, they are said to occur spontaneously. Exergonic reactions are considered spontaneous because they result in a negative delta G ($-\Delta$G), where the products of the reaction have less free energy within them than the reactants. Endergonic reactions require an input of energy and result in a positive delta G ($+\Delta$G), with the products of the reaction containing more free energy than the individual reactants. When a system no longer has free energy to do work, it has reached **equilibrium**. Since cells always work, they are no longer alive if they reach equilibrium.

Cells balance their energy resources by using the energy from exergonic reactions to drive endergonic reactions forward, a process called **energy coupling**. **Adenosine triphosphate**, or ATP, is a molecule that is an immediate source of energy for cellular work. When it is broken down, it releases energy used in endergonic reactions and anabolic pathways. ATP breaks down into adenosine diphosphate, or ADP, and a separate phosphate group, releasing energy in an exergonic reaction. As ATP is used up by reactions, it is also regenerated by having a new phosphate group added onto the ADP products within the cell in an endergonic reaction.

Enzymes are special proteins that help speed up metabolic reactions and pathways. They do not change the overall free energy release or consumption of reactions; they just make the reactions occur more quickly as it lowers the activation energy required. Enzymes are designed to act only on specific substrates. Their physical shape fits snugly onto their matched substrates, so enzymes only speed up reactions that contain the substrates to which they are matched.

The Cell

Cells are the basic structural and functional unit of all organisms. They are the smallest unit of matter that is living. While there are many single-celled organisms, most biological organisms are more complex and made up of many different types of cells. There are two distinct types of cells: prokaryotic and eukaryotic. **Prokaryotic cells** include bacteria, while **eukaryotic cells** include animal and plant cells. Both types of cells are enclosed by a **cell membrane**, which is selectively permeable. Selective permeability means essentially that it is a gatekeeper, allowing certain molecules and ions in and out, and keeping unwanted ones at bay, at least until they are ready for use. Both contain ribosomes, which are complexes that make protein inside the cell, and DNA. One major difference is that the DNA in eukaryotic cells are enclosed in a membrane-bound **nucleus**, where in prokaryotic cells, DNA is in the **nucleoid**, a region that is not enclosed by a membrane. Another major difference is that eukaryotic cells contain **organelles,** which are membrane-enclosed structures, each with a specific function, while prokaryotic cells do not have organelles.

Organelles Found in Eukaryotic Cells

The following cell organelles are found in both animal and plant cells unless otherwise noted:

Nucleus: The nucleus consists of three parts: nuclear envelope, nucleolus, and chromatin. The **nuclear envelope** is the double membrane that surrounds the nucleus and separates its contents from the rest of the cell. It is porous so substances can pass back and forth between the nucleus and the other parts of the cell. It is also continuous, with the endoplasmic reticulum that is present within the cytosol of the cell. The **nucleolus** is in charge of producing ribosomes. **Chromosomes** are comprised of tightly coiled proteins, RNA, and DNA and are collectively called **chromatin**.

Endoplasmic Reticulum (ER): The ER is a network of membranous sacs and tubes responsible for membrane synthesis and other metabolic and synthetic activities of the cell. There are two types of ER, rough and smooth. **Rough ER** is lined with ribosomes and is the location of protein synthesis. This provides a separate compartment for site-specific protein synthesis and is important for the intracellular transport of proteins. **Smooth ER** does not contain ribosomes and is the location of lipid synthesis.

Flagellum: The flagellum is found in protists and animal cells. It is a cluster of microtubules projected out of the plasma membrane and aids in cell motility.

Centrosome: The centrosome is the area of the cell where microtubules are created and organized for mitosis. Each centrosome contains two **centrioles.**

Cytoskeleton: The cytoskeleton in animal cells is made up of microfilaments, intermediate filaments, and microtubules. In plant cells, the cytoskeleton is made up of only microfilaments and microtubules. These structures reinforce the cell's shape and aid in cell movements.

Microvilli: Microvilli are found only in animal cells. They are protrusions in the cell membrane that increase the cell's surface area. They have a variety of functions, including absorption, secretion, and cellular adhesion.

Peroxisome: A peroxisome contains enzymes that are involved in many of the cell's metabolic functions, one of the most important being the breakdown of fatty acid chains. It produces hydrogen peroxide as a by-product of these processes and then converts the hydrogen peroxide to water.

Mitochondrion: The mitochondrion, considered the cell's powerhouse, is one of the most important structures for maintaining regular cell function. It is where cellular respiration occurs and where most of the cell's ATP is generated.

Lysosome: Lysosomes are found exclusively in animal cells. They are responsible for digestion and can hydrolyze macromolecules.

Golgi Apparatus: The Golgi apparatus is responsible for synthesizing, modifying, sorting, transporting, and secreting cell products. Because of its large size, it was one of the first organelles studied in detail.

Ribosomes: Ribosomes are found either free in the cytosol, bound to the rough ER, or bound to the nuclear envelope. They are also found in prokaryotes. Ribosomes make up a complex that forms proteins within the cell.

Plasmodesmata: Found only in plant cells, plasmodesmata are cytoplasmic channels, or tunnels, that go through the cell wall and connect the cytoplasm of adjacent cells.

Chloroplast: Chloroplasts are plastids found in protists, such as algae and plant cells. It is responsible for photosynthesis, which is the process of converting sunlight to chemical energy that is stored and used later to drive cellular activities.

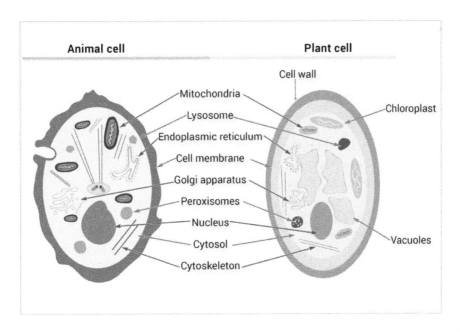

Vacuoles: Vacuoles are membrane-bound organelles found primarily in plant and fungi cells, but also in some animal cells. Vacuoles are filled with water and some enzymes and are important for intracellular digestion and waste removal. The membrane-bound nature of the vacuole allows for the storage of harmful material and poisonous substances. The pressure from the water inside the vacuole also contributes to the structure of plant cells. Animals have food vacuoles that contain the contents of phagocytosis. **Phagocytosis**, or "cellular eating," occurs when a cell engulfs large particles and internalizes them by using vacuoles.

Central Vacuole: A central vacuole is found only in plant cells, and is responsible for storage, breakdown of waste products, and hydrolysis of macromolecules.

Plasma Membrane: The plasma membrane is a phospholipid bilayer that encloses the cell. It is also found in prokaryotes.

Cell Wall: Cell walls are present in fungi, plant cells, and some protists. The cell wall is made up of strong fibrous substances, including cellulose (plants), chitin (fungi) and other polysaccharides, and protein. It is a layer outside of the plasma membrane that protects the cell from mechanical damage and helps maintain the cell's shape.

Cellular Respiration

Cellular respiration is a set of metabolic processes that converts energy from nutrients into ATP. Respiration can either occur aerobically, using oxygen, or anaerobically, without oxygen. While prokaryotic cells carry out respiration in the cytosol, most of the respiration in eukaryotic cells occurs in the mitochondria.

Aerobic Respiration

There are three main steps in aerobic cellular respiration: glycolysis, the citric acid cycle (also known as the Krebs cycle), and oxidative phosphorylation. **Glycolysis** is an essential metabolic pathway that converts glucose to pyruvate and allows for cellular respiration to occur. It does not require oxygen to be present. Glucose is a common molecule used for energy production in cells. During glycolysis, two three-carbon sugars are generated from the splitting of a glucose molecule. These smaller sugars are then converted into pyruvate molecules via oxidation and atom rearrangement. Glycolysis requires two ATP molecules to drive the process forward, but the end product of the process has four ATP molecules, for a net production of two ATP molecules. Also, two reduced nicotinamide adenine dinucleotide (NADH) molecules are created from when the electron carrier oxidized nicotinamide adenine dinucleotide (NAD+) peels off two electrons and a hydrogen atom.

In aerobically-respiring eukaryotic cells, the pyruvate molecules then enter the mitochondrion. Pyruvate is oxidized and converted into a compound called acetyl-CoA. This molecule enters the **citric acid cycle** to begin the process of aerobic respiration.

The citric acid cycle has eight steps. Remember that glycolysis produces two pyruvate molecules from each glucose molecule. Each pyruvate molecule oxidizes into a single acetyl-CoA molecule, which then enters the citric acid cycle. Therefore, two citric acid cycles can be completed and twice the number of ATP molecules are generated per glucose molecule.

Eight Steps of the Citric Acid Cycle

Step 1: Acetyl-CoA adds a two-carbon acetyl group to an oxaloacetate molecule and produces one citrate molecule.

Step 2: Citrate is converted to its isomer isocitrate by removing one water molecule and adding a new water molecule in a different configuration.

Step 3: Isocitrate is oxidized and converted to α-ketoglutarate. A carbon dioxide (CO_2) molecule is released and one NAD+ molecule is converted to NADH.

Step 4: α-Ketoglutarate is converted to succinyl-CoA. Another carbon dioxide molecule is released and another NAD+ molecule is converted to NADH.

Step 5: Succinyl-CoA becomes succinate by the addition of a phosphate group to the cycle. The oxygen molecule of the phosphate group attaches to the succinyl-CoA molecule and the CoA group is released. The rest of the phosphate group transfers to a guanosine diphosphate (GDP) molecule, converting it to guanosine triphosphate (GTP). GTP acts similarly to ATP and can actually be used to generate an ATP molecule at this step.

Step 6: Succinate is converted to fumarate by losing two hydrogen atoms. The hydrogen atoms join a flavin adenine dinucleotide (FAD) molecule, converting it to $FADH_2$, which is a hydroquinone form.

Step 7: A water molecule is added to the cycle and converts fumarate to malate.

Step 8: Malate is oxidized and converted to oxaloacetate. One lost hydrogen atom is added to an NAD molecule to create NADH. The oxaloacetate generated here then enters back into step one of the cycle.

At the end of glycolysis and the citric acid cycles, four ATP molecules have been generated. The NADH and FADH$_2$ molecules are used as energy to drive the next step of oxidative phosphorylation.

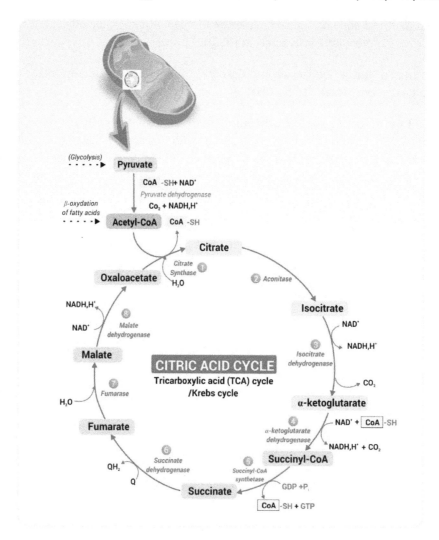

Oxidative Phosphorylation

Oxidative phosphorylation includes two steps: the electron transport chain and chemiosmosis. The inner mitochondrial membrane has four protein complexes, sequenced I to IV, used to transport protons and electrons through the inner mitochondrial matrix. Two electrons and a proton (H+) are passed from each NADH and FADH$_2$ to these channel proteins, pumping the hydrogen ions to the inner-membrane space using energy from the high-energy electrons to create a concentration gradient. NADH and FADH$_2$ also drop their high-energy electrons to the electron transport chain. NAD+ and FAD molecules in the mitochondrial matrix return to the Krebs cycle to pick up materials for the next delivery. From here, two processes happen simultaneously:

1. **Electron Transport Chain:** In addition to complexes I to IV, there are two mobile electron carriers present in the inner mitochondrial membrane, called **ubiquinone** and **cytochrome C.** At the end of this transport chain, electrons are accepted by an O$_2$ molecule in the matrix, and water is formed with the addition of two hydrogen atoms from chemiosmosis.

2. **Chemiosmosis:** This occurs in an ATP synthase complex that sits next to the four electron transporting complexes. ATP synthase uses **facilitated diffusion** (passive transport) to deliver protons across the concentration gradient from the inner mitochondrial membrane to the matrix. As the protons travel, the ATP synthase protein physically spins, and the kinetic energy generated is invested into phosphorylation of ADP molecules to generate ATP. Oxidative phosphorylation produces twenty-six to twenty-eight ATP molecules, bringing the total number of ATP generated through glycolysis and cellular respiration to thirty to thirty-two molecules.

Anaerobic Respiration

Some organisms do not live in oxygen-rich environments and must find alternate methods of respiration. Anaerobic respiration occurs in certain prokaryotic organisms. They utilize an electron transport chain similar to the aerobic respiration pathway; however, the terminal acceptor molecule is an electronegative substance that is not O_2. Some bacteria, for example, use the sulfate ion (SO_4^{2-}) as the final electron accepting molecule and the resulting byproduct is hydrogen sulfide (H_2S) instead of water.

Muscle cells that reach anaerobic threshold go through lactic acid respiration, while yeasts go through alcohol fermentation. Both processes only make two ATP.

Photosynthesis

Photosynthesis is the process of converting light energy into chemical energy that is then stored in sugar and other organic molecules. It can be divided into two stages: the light-dependent reactions and the Calvin cycle. In plants, the photosynthetic process takes place in the chloroplast. Inside the chloroplast are membranous sacs, called **thylakoids**. Chlorophyll is a green pigment that lives in the thylakoid membranes and absorbs the light energy, starting the process of photosynthesis. The **Calvin cycle** takes place in the **stroma,** or inner space, of the chloroplasts. The complex series of reactions that take place in photosynthesis can be simplified into the following equation: $6CO_2 + 12H_2O +$ Light Energy $\rightarrow C_6H_{12}O_6 + 6O_2 + 6H_2O$. Basically, carbon dioxide and water mix with light energy inside the chloroplast to produce organic molecules, oxygen, and water. Note that water is on both sides of the equation. Twelve water molecules are consumed during this process and six water molecules are newly formed as byproducts.

The Light Reactions

During the **light reactions**, chlorophyll molecules absorb light energy, or solar energy. In the thylakoid membrane, chlorophyll molecules, together with other small molecules and proteins, form photosystems, which are made up of a reaction-center complex surrounded by a light-harvesting complex. In the first step of photosynthesis, the light-harvesting complex from photosystem II (PSII) absorbs a photon from light, passes the photon from one pigment molecule to another within itself, and then transfers it to the reaction-center complex. Inside the reaction-center complex, the energy from the photon enables a special pair of chlorophyll *a* molecules to release two electrons. These two electrons are then accepted by a primary electron acceptor molecule. Simultaneously, a water molecule is split into two hydrogen atoms, two electrons and one oxygen atom. The two electrons are transferred one by one to the chlorophyll *a* molecules, replacing their released electrons. The released electrons are then transported down an electron transport chain by attaching to the electron carrier plastoquinone (Pq), a cytochrome complex, and then a protein called plastocyanin (Pc) before they reach photosystem I (PS I). As the electrons pass through the cytochrome complex, protons are pumped into the thylakoid space, providing the concentration gradient that will eventually travel through ATP synthase to make

ATP (like in aerobic respiration). PS I absorbs photons from light, similar to PS II. However, the electrons that are released from the chlorophyll *a* molecules in PS I are replaced by the electrons coming down the electron transport chain (from PS II). A primary electron acceptor molecule accepts the released electrons in PS I and passes the electrons onto another electron transport chain involving the protein ferredoxin (Fd). In the final steps of the light reactions, electrons are transferred from Fd to Nicotinamide adenine dinucleotide phosphate (NADP+) with the help of the enzyme NADP+ reductase and NADPH is produced. The ATP and nicotinamide adenine dinucleotide phosphate-oxidase (NADPH) produced from the light reactions are used as energy to form organic molecules in the Calvin cycle.

The Calvin Cycle

There are three phases in the Calvin cycle: carbon fixation, reduction, and regeneration of the CO_2 acceptor. **Carbon fixation** is when the first carbon molecule is introduced into the cycle, when CO_2 from the air is absorbed by the chloroplast. Each CO_2 molecule enters the cycle and attaches to ribulose bisphosphate (RuBP), a five-carbon sugar. The enzyme RuBP carboxylase-oxygenase, also known as rubisco, catalyzes this reaction. Next, two three-carbon 3-phosphoglycerate sugar molecules are formed immediately from the splitting of the six-carbon sugar.

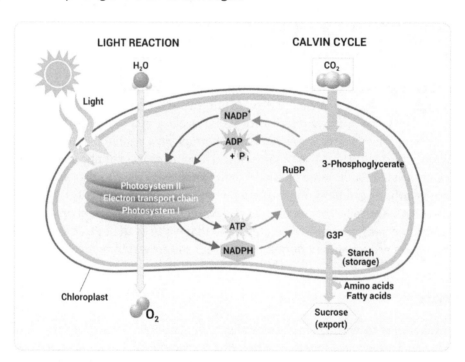

Next, during the **reduction** phase, an ATP molecule is reduced to ADP and the phosphate group attaches to 3-phosphoglycerate, forming 1,3-bisphosphoglycerate. An NADPH molecule then donates two high-energy electrons to the newly formed 1,3-bisphosphate, causing it to lose the phosphate group and become glyceraldehyde 3-phosphate (G3P), which is a high-energy sugar molecule. At this point in the cycle, one G3P molecule exits the cycle and is used by the plant. However, to regenerate RuBP molecules, which are the CO_2 acceptors in the cycle, five G3P molecules continue in the cycle. It takes three turns of the cycle and three CO_2 molecules entering the cycle to form one G3P molecule.

In the final phase of the Calvin cycle, three RuBP molecules are formed from the rearrangement of the carbon skeletons of five G3P molecules. It is a complex process that involves the reduction of three ATP

162

molecules. At the end of the process, RuBP molecules are again ready to enter the first phase and accept CO_2 molecules.

Although the Calvin cycle is not dependent on light energy, both steps of photosynthesis usually occur during daylight, as the Calvin cycle is dependent upon the ATP and NADPH produced by the light reactions, because that energy can be invested into bonds to create high-energy sugars. The Calvin cycle invests nine ATP molecules and six NADPH molecules into every one molecule of G3P that it produces. The G3P that is produced can be used as the starting material to build larger organic compounds, such as glucose.

Cellular Reproduction

Cellular reproduction is the process that cells use to divide into two new cells. The ability of a multi-cellular organism to generate new cells to replace dying and damaged cells is vital for sustaining its life. Bacteria reproduce via **binary fission**, which is a simpler process than eukaryotic division because it doesn't involve splitting a nucleus and doesn't have a web of proteins to pull chromosomes apart. Bacteria copy their DNA in a process called DNA replication, grow, and then the replicated DNA moves to either side, and two new cells are made.

There are two processes by which a eukaryotic cell can divide: mitosis and meiosis. In **mitosis,** the daughter cells produced from parental cell division are identical to each other and the parent. **Meiosis** produces genetically unique haploid cells due to two stages of cell division. Meiosis produces **haploid** cells, or **gametes** (sperm and egg cells), which only have one set of chromosomes. Humans are **diploid** because we have two sets of chromosomes – one from each parent. **Somatic** (body) cells are all diploid and are produced via mitosis.

Mitosis

Mitosis is the division of the genetic material in the nucleus of a cell, and is immediately followed by **cytokinesis**, which is the division of the cytoplasm of the cell. The two processes make up the mitotic phase of the cell cycle. Mitosis can be broken down into five stages: prophase, prometaphase, metaphase, anaphase, and telophase. Mitosis is preceded by **interphase**, where the cell spends the majority of its life while growing and replicating its DNA.

Prophase: During this phase, the mitotic spindles begin to form. They are made up of centrosomes and microtubules. As the microtubules lengthen, the centrosomes move farther away from each other. The nucleolus disappears and the chromatin fibers begin to coil up and form chromosomes. Two sister **chromatids**, which are two identical copies of one chromosome, are joined together at the centromere.

Prometaphase: The nuclear envelope begins to break down and the microtubules enter the nuclear area. Each pair of chromatin fibers develops a **kinetochore**, which is a specialized protein structure in the middle of the adjoined fibers. The chromosomes are further condensed.

Metaphase: The microtubules are stretched across the cell and the centrosomes are at opposite ends of the cell. The chromosomes align at the **metaphase plate**, which is a plane that is exactly between the two centrosomes. The centromere of each chromosome is attached to the kinetochore microtubules that are stretching from each centrosome to the metaphase plate.

Anaphase: The sister chromatids break apart, forming individual chromosomes. The two daughter chromosomes move to opposite ends of the cell. The microtubules shorten toward opposite ends of the cell as well. The cell elongates and, by the end of this phase, there is a complete set of chromosomes at each end of the cell.

Telophase: Two nuclei form at each end of the cell and nuclear envelopes begin to form around each nucleus. The nucleoli reappear and the chromosomes become less condensed. The microtubules are broken down by the cell and mitosis is complete.

Cytokinesis divides the cytoplasm by pinching off the cytoplasm, forming a cleavage furrow, and the two daughter cells then enter interphase, completing the cycle.

Plant cell mitosis is similar except that it lacks centromeres, and instead has a microtubule organizing center. Cytokinesis occurs with the formation of a cell plate.

Meiosis

Meiosis is a type of cell division in which the parent cell has twice as many sets of chromosomes as the daughter cells into which it divides. Although the first stage of meiosis involves the duplication of chromosomes, similar to that of mitosis, the parent cell in meiosis divides into four cells, as opposed to the two produced in mitosis.

Meiosis has the same phases as mitosis, except that they occur twice: once in meiosis I and again in meiosis II. The diploid parent has two sets of homologous chromosomes, one set from each parent. During meiosis I, each chromosome set goes through a process called **crossing over**, which jumbles up the genes on each chromatid. In anaphase one, the separated chromosomes are no longer identical and, once the chromosomes pull apart, each daughter cell is haploid (one set of chromosomes with two non-identical sister chromatids). Next, during meiosis II, the two intermediate daughter cells divide again, separating the chromatids, producing a total of four total haploid cells that each contains one set of chromosomes.

Genetics

Genetics is the study of heredity, which is the transmission of traits from one generation to the next, and hereditary variation. The chromosomes passed from parent to child contain hereditary information in the form of genes. Each gene has specific sequences of DNA that encode proteins, start pathways, and result in inherited traits. In the human life cycle, one haploid sperm cell joins one haploid egg cell to form a diploid cell. The diploid cell is the zygote, the first cell of the new organism, and from then on mitosis takes over and nine months later, there is a fully developed human that has billions of identical cells.

The monk Gregor Mendel is referred to as the father of genetics. In the 1860s, Mendel came up with one of the first models of inheritance, using peapods with different traits in the garden at his abbey to test his theory and develop his model. His model included three laws to determine which traits are inherited; his theories still apply today, after genetics has been studied more in depth.

1. The **Law of Dominance:** Each characteristic has two versions that can be inherited. The gene that encodes for the characteristic has two variations, or alleles, and one is dominant over the other.

2. The **Law of Segregation:** When two parent cells form daughter cells, the alleles segregate and each daughter cell only inherits one of the alleles from each parent.

3. The **Law of Independent Assortment:** Different traits are inherited independent of one another because in metaphase, the set of chromosomes line up in random fashion – mom's set of chromosomes do not line up all on the left or right, there is a random mix.

Organisms contain a **genotype** and a **phenotype**. The genotype is the DNA present in the cells that code for the genes, and the phenotype is the set of observable traits that are expressed. For example, a brown-eyed girl may have genes for both blue and brown eyes, but the actual physical trait expressed is brown eyes. So, the genotype is blue and brown eyes, but the phenotype is brown eyes.

Dominant and Recessive Traits

Each gene has two **alleles**, one inherited from each parent. **Dominant alleles** are noted in capital letters (A) and **recessive alleles** are noted in lower case letters (a). There are three possible combinations of alleles among dominant and recessive alleles: AA, Aa, and aa. If both alleles are identical, the individual is considered **homozygous**; if the two alleles have different sequences, the individual is considered **heterozygous**. In most genes, one allele is considered more dominant than the other and will mask the appearance of the less dominant, or recessive, allele when there is a heterozygous situation. Dominant alleles, when mixed with recessive alleles, will mask the recessive trait. The recessive trait would only appear as the phenotype when the allele combination is aa because a dominant allele is not present to mask it.

Although most genes follow the standard dominant/recessive rules, there are some genes that defy them. Examples include cases of co-dominance, multiple alleles, incomplete dominance, sex-linked traits, and polygenic inheritance.

In cases of **co-dominance**, both alleles are expressed equally. For example, blood type has three alleles: I^A, I^B, and i. I^A and I^B are both dominant to i, but co-dominant with each other. An $I^A I^B$ has AB blood. With incomplete dominance, the allele combination Aa actually makes a third phenotype. An example: certain flowers can be red (AA), white (aa), or pink (Aa).

Punnett Square

For simple genetic combinations, a **Punnett square** can be used to assess the phenotypes of subsequent generations. In a 2 x 2 cell square, one parent's alleles are set up in columns and the other parent's alleles are in rows. The resulting allele combinations are shown in the four internal cells.

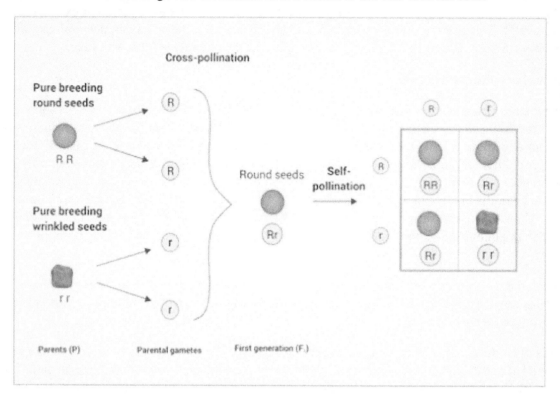

In the example above, two parents with alleles RR and rr, have a 50% chance (2 in 4) of having an offspring with alleles Rr.

Mutations

Genetic **mutations** occur when there is a permanent alteration in the DNA sequence that codes for a specific gene. They can be small, affecting only one base pair, or large, affecting many genes on a chromosome. Mutations are classified as either hereditary, which means they were also present in the parent gene, or acquired, meaning they occurred after the genes were passed down from the parents. Although mutations are not common, they are an important aspect of genetics and variation in the general population.

DNA

DNA is made of nucleotide, and contains the genetic information of a living organism. It consists of two polynucleotide strands that are twisted and linked together in a double-helix structure. The polynucleotide strands are made up of four nitrogenous bases: adenine (A), thymine (T), guanine (G), and cytosine (C). Adenine and guanine are purines while thymine and cytosine are pyrimidines. These bases have specific pairings of A with T, and G with C. The bases are ordered so that these specific pairings will occur when the two polynucleotide strands coil together to form a DNA molecule. The two strands of DNA are described as antiparallel because one strand runs 5' $\rightarrow$ 3' while the other strand of the helix runs 3' $\rightarrow$ 5'.

Before chromosome replication and cell division can occur, DNA replication must happen in interphase. There are specific base pair sequences on DNA, called origins of replication, where DNA replication begins. The proteins that begin the replication process attach to this site and begin separating the two strands and creating a replication bubble. Each end of the bubble has a replication fork, which is a Y-shaped area of the DNA that is being unwound. Several types of proteins are important to the beginning of DNA replication. **Helicases** are enzymes responsible for untwisting the two strands at the replication fork. Single-strand binding proteins bind to the separated strands so that they do not join back together during the replication process. While part of the DNA is unwound, the remainder of the molecule becomes even more twisted in response. Topoisomerase enzymes help relieve this strain by breaking, untwisting, and rejoining the DNA strands.

Once the DNA strand is unwound, an initial primer chain of RNA from the enzyme primase is made to start replication. Replication of DNA can only occur in the 5' → 3' direction. Therefore, during replication, one strand of the DNA template creates the leading strand in the 5' → 3' direction and the other strand creates the lagging strand. While the leading strand is created efficiently and in one piece, the lagging strand is generated in fragments, called **Okazaki fragments**, then are pieced together to form a complete strand by DNA ligase. Following the primer chain of RNA, DNA polymerases are the enzymes responsible for extending the DNA chains by adding on base pairs.

DNA forms the genetic code in the nucleus of eukaryotes, and RNA is the interpreter that comes in many varieties.

- **Messenger RNA (mRNA)** copies the DNA into a complementary transcript. This process is called **transcription**.

- **Ribosomal RNA (rRNA)** makes up the protein-making structure called the ribosome which reads the transcript in a process called **translation.**

Transfer RNA (tRNA) carries amino acids and delivers them to the ribosome. Each three letters of the mRNA transcript, or **codon**, recruits the anti-codon of a tRNA molecule that carries the corresponding amino acid. Only when a **stop codon** is reached will the ribosome disassemble, thus releasing the assembled protein.

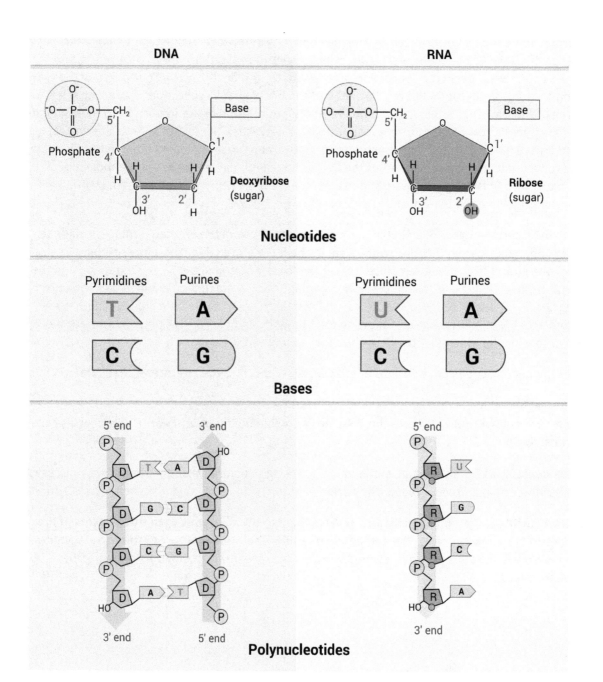

Nucleotides

DNA

RNA

Bases

Pyrimidines · Purines

Polynucleotides

Practice Questions

1. A scientist is trying to determine how much poison will kill a rat the fastest. Which of the following statements is an example of an appropriate hypothesis?
    a. Rats that are given lots of poison seem to die quickly.
    b. Does the amount of poison affect how quickly the rat dies?
    c. The more poison a rat is given, the quicker it will die.
    d. Poison is fatal to rats.

2. Which of the following is NOT a unique property of water?
    a. High cohesion and adhesion
    b. High surface tension
    c. High density upon melting
    d. High freezing point

3. What is a metabolic reaction that releases energy called?
    a. Catabolic
    b. Carbolic
    c. Anabolic
    d. Endothermic

4. What organic compounds facilitate chemical reactions by lowering activation energy?
    a. Carbohydrates
    b. Lipids
    c. Enzymes
    d. Nucleotides

5. Which structure is exclusively in eukaryotic cells?
    a. Cell wall
    b. Nucleus
    c. Cell membrane
    d. Vacuole

6. Which of these is NOT found in the cell nucleus?
    a. Golgi complex
    b. Chromosomes
    c. Nucleolus
    d. Chromatin

7. Which is the cellular organelle used for digestion to recycle materials?
    a. Golgi apparatus
    b. Lysosome
    c. Centriole
    d. Mitochondria

8. What are the energy-generating structures of the cell called?
   a. Nucleoplasms
   b. Mitochondria
   c. Golgi Apparatus
   d. Ribosomes

9. Which is a component of plant cells not found in animal cells?
   a. Nucleus
   b. Plastid
   c. Cell membrane
   d. Lysosome

10. What is the LAST phase of mitosis?
    a. Prophase
    b. Telophase
    c. Anaphase
    d. Metaphase

11. How many daughter cells are formed from one parent cell during meiosis?
    a. One
    b. Two
    c. Three
    d. Four

12. Which of the choices below are the reproductive cells produced by meiosis?
    a. Genes
    b. Alleles
    c. Chromatids
    d. Gametes

13. What is the process of cell division in somatic (most body) cells called?
    a. Mitosis
    b. Meiosis
    c. Respiration
    d. Cytogenesis

14. What type of biological molecule is a monosaccharide?
    a. Protein
    b. Nucleic acid
    c. Carbohydrate
    d. Lipid

15. With which genotype would the recessive phenotype appear, if the dominant allele is marked with "A" and the recessive allele is marked with "a"?
    a. AA
    b. aa
    c. Aa
    d. aA

16. What is an alteration in the normal gene sequence called?
    a. Mutation
    b. Gene migration
    c. Polygenetic inheritance
    d. Incomplete dominance

17. Blood type is a trait determined by multiple alleles, and two of them are co-dominant: I^A codes for A blood and I^B codes for B blood. i codes for O blood and is recessive to both. If an A heterozygote individual and an O individual have a child, what is the probably that the child will have A blood?
    a. 25%
    b. 50%
    c. 75%
    d. 100%

18. What are the building blocks of DNA referred to as?
    a. Helices
    b. Proteins
    c. Genes
    d. Nucleotides

19. Which statement is NOT true about DNA?
    a. It has guanine.
    b. DNA enables living organisms to pass on their genetic information.
    c. It can be single-stranded.
    d. DNA replication happens in interphase.

20. Which of the following is true about an endergonic reaction?
    a. The reaction results in a negative delta G ($-\Delta G$).
    b. The reaction is considered spontaneous.
    c. The reaction absorbs energy.
    d. The reaction releases energy.

21. What is the term used for the set of metabolic reactions that convert chemical bonds to energy in the form of ATP?
    a. Photosynthesis
    b. Reproduction
    c. Active transport
    d. Cellular respiration

22. Which level of protein structure is defined by the folds and coils of the protein's polypeptide backbone?
    a. Primary
    b. Secondary
    c. Tertiary
    d. Quaternary

23. What is the broadest, or LEAST specialized, classification of the Linnean taxonomic system?
    a. Species
    b. Family
    c. Domain
    d. Phylum

24. Which of the following is NOT a function of lipids?
    a. Provides cellular instructions
    b. Can be chemical messages
    c. Provides energy
    d. Composes cell membranes

25. What is the cell structure responsible for protein synthesis called?
    a. DNA
    b. Golgi Apparatus
    c. Nucleus
    d. Ribosome

Answer Explanations

1. C: A hypothesis is a statement that makes a prediction between two variables. The two variables here are the amount of poison and how quickly the rat dies. Choice C states that the more poison a rat is given, the more quickly it will die, which is a prediction. Choice A is incorrect because it's simply an observation. Choice B is incorrect because it's a question posed by the observation but makes no predictions. Choice D is incorrect because it's simply a fact.

2. D: Water's unique properties are due to intermolecular hydrogen bonding. These forces make water molecules "stick" to one another, which explains why water has unusually high cohesion and adhesion (sticking to each other and sticking to other surfaces). Cohesion can be seen in beads of dew. Adhesion can be seen when water sticks to the sides of a graduated cylinder to form a meniscus. The stickiness to neighboring molecules also increases surface tension, providing a very thin film that light things cannot penetrate, which is observed when leaves float in swimming pools. Water has a low freezing point, not a high freezing point, due to the fact that molecules have to have a very low kinetic energy to arrange themselves in the lattice-like structure found in ice, its solid form.

3. A: Catabolic reactions release energy and are exothermic. Catabolism breaks down complex molecules into simpler molecules. Anabolic reactions are just the opposite—they absorb energy in order to form complex molecules from simpler ones. Proteins, carbohydrates (polysaccharides), lipids, and nucleic acids are complex organic molecules synthesized by anabolic metabolism. The monomers of these organic compounds are amino acids, monosaccharides, triglycerides, and nucleotides.

4. C: Metabolic reactions utilize enzymes to decrease their activation energy. Enzymes that drive these reactions are protein catalysts. Their mechanism is sometimes referred to as the "lock-and-key" model. "Lock and key" references the fact that enzymes have exact specificity with their substrate (reactant) like a lock does to a key. The substrate binds to the enzyme snugly, the enzyme facilitates the reaction, and then product is formed while the enzyme is unchanged and ready to be reused.

5. B: The structure exclusively found in eukaryotic cells is the nucleus. Animal, plant, fungi, and protist cells are all eukaryotic. DNA is contained within the nucleus of eukaryotic cells, and they also have membrane-bound organelles that perform complex intracellular metabolic activities. Prokaryotic cells (archae and bacteria) do not have a nucleus or other membrane-bound organelles and are less complex than eukaryotic cells.

6. A:. The Golgi complex, also known as the Golgi apparatus, is not found in the nucleus. Chromosomes, the nucleolus, and chromatin are all found within the nucleus of the cell. The Golgi apparatus is found in the cytoplasm and is responsible for protein maturation, the process of proteins folding into their secondary, tertiary, and quaternary configurations. The structure appears folded in membranous layers and is easily visible with microscopy. The Golgi apparatus packages proteins in vesicles for export out of the cell or to their cellular destination.

7. B: The cell structure responsible for cellular storage, digestion, and waste removal is the lysosome. Lysosomes are like recycle bins. They are filled with digestive enzymes that facilitate catabolic reactions to regenerate monomers.

8. B: The mitochondria are cellular energy generators and the "powerhouses" of the cell. They provide cellular energy in the form of adenosine triphosphate (ATP). This process, called aerobic respiration, uses oxygen plus sugars, proteins, and fats to produce ATP, carbon dioxide, and water. Mitochondria contain their own DNA and ribosomes, which is significant because according to endosymbiotic theory, these structures provide evidence that they used to be independently-functioning prokaryotes.

9. B: Plastids are the photosynthesizing organelles of plants that are not found in animal cells. Plants have the ability to generate their own sugars through photosynthesis, a process where they use pigments to capture the sun's light energy. Chloroplasts are the most prevalent plastid, and chlorophyll is the light-absorbing pigment that absorbs all energy carried in photons except that of green light. This explains why the photosynthesizing parts of plants, predominantly leaves, appear green.

10. B: During telophase, two nuclei form at each end of the cell and nuclear envelopes begin to form around each nucleus. The nucleoli reappear, and the chromosomes become less compact. The microtubules are broken down by the cell, and mitosis is complete. The process begins with prophase as the mitotic spindles begin to form from centrosomes. Prometaphase follows, with the breakdown of the nuclear envelope and the further condensing of the chromosomes. Next, metaphase occurs when the microtubules are stretched across the cell and the chromosomes align at the metaphase plate. Finally, in the last step before telophase, anaphase occurs as the sister chromatids break apart and form chromosomes.

11. D: Meiosis has the same phases as mitosis, except that they occur twice—once in meiosis I and once in meiosis II. During meiosis I, the cell splits into two. Each cell contains two sets of chromosomes. Next, during meiosis II, the two intermediate daughter cells divide again, producing four total haploid cells that each contain one set of chromosomes.

12. D: Reproductive cells are referred to as gametes: egg (female) and sperm (male). These cells have only 1 set of 23 chromosomes and are haploid so that when they combine during fertilization, the zygote has the correct diploid number, 46. Reproductive cell division is called meiosis, which is different from mitosis, the type of division process for body (somatic) cells.

13. A: The process of cell division in somatic is mitosis. In interphase, which precedes mitosis, cells prepare for division by copying their DNA. Once mitotic machinery has been assembled in interphase, mitosis occurs, which has four distinct phases: prophase, metaphase, anaphase, and telophase, followed by cytokinesis, which is the final splitting of the cytoplasm. The two diploid daughter cells are genetically identical to the parent cell.

14. C: Carbohydrates consist of sugars. The simplest sugar molecule is called a monosaccharide and has the molecular formula of CH_2O, or a multiple of that formula. Monosaccharides are important molecules for cellular respiration. Their carbon skeleton can also be used to rebuild new small molecules. Lipids are fats, proteins are formed via amino acids, and nucleic acid is found in DNA and RNA.

15. B: Dominant alleles are considered to have stronger phenotypes and, when mixed with recessive alleles, will mask the recessive trait. The recessive trait would only appear as the phenotype when the allele combination is "aa" because a dominant allele is not present to mask it.

16. A: An alteration in the normal gene sequence is called a DNA point mutation. Mutations can be harmful, neutral, or even beneficial. Sometimes, as seen in natural selection, a genetic mutation can improve fitness, providing an adaptation that will aid in survival. DNA mutations can happen as a result of environmental damage, for example, from radiation or chemicals. Mutations can also happen during cell replication, as a result of incorrect pairing of complementary nucleotides by DNA polymerase. There are also chromosomal mutations as well, where entire segments of chromosomes can be deleted, inverted, duplicated, or sent or received from a different chromosome.

17. B: 50%. According to the Punnett square, the child has a 2 out of 4 chance of having A-type blood, since the dominant allele I^A is present in two of the four possible offspring. The O-type blood allele is masked by the A-type blood allele since it is recessive.

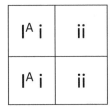

I^A i	ii
I^A i	ii

18. D: The building blocks of DNA are nucleotides. A nucleotide is a five-carbon sugar with a phosphate group and a nitrogenous base (Adenine, Guanine, Cytosine, and Thymine). DNA is a double helix and looks like a spiral ladder. Each side has a sugar/phosphate backbone, and the rungs of the ladder that connect the sides are the nitrogen bases. Adenine always pairs with thymine via two hydrogen bonds, and cytosine always pairs with guanine via three hydrogen bonds. The weak hydrogen bonds are important because they allow DNA to easily be opened for replication and transcription.

19. C: DNA is made of nucleotide and contains the genetic information of a living organism. It consists of two polynucleotide strands that are twisted and linked together in a double-helix structure. RNA is made up of a single strand of nucleotides that folds onto itself.

20. C: Endergonic reactions absorb free energy from its surroundings. Answer choices A, B, and D are all qualities of exergonic reactions.

21. D: Cellular respiration is the term used for the set of metabolic reactions that convert chemical bonds to energy in the form of ATP. All respiration starts with glycolysis in the cytoplasm, and in the presence of oxygen, the process will continue to the mitochondria. In a series of oxidation/reduction reactions, primarily glucose will be broken down so that the energy contained within its bonds can be transferred to the smaller ATP molecules. It's like having a $100 bill (glucose) as opposed to having one hundred $1 bills. This is beneficial to the organism because it allows energy to be distributed throughout the cell very easily in smaller packets of energy.

When glucose is broken down, its electrons and hydrogen atoms are involved in oxidative phosphorylation in order to make ATP, while its carbon and oxygen atoms are released as carbon dioxide. Anaerobic respiration does not occur frequently in humans, but during rigorous exercise, lack of available oxygen in the muscles can lead to anaerobic ATP production in a process called lactic acid fermentation. Alcohol fermentation is another type of anaerobic respiration that occurs in yeast. Anaerobic respiration is extremely less efficient than aerobic respiration, as it has a net yield of 2ATP, while aerobic respiration's net yield exceeds 30 ATP.

22. C: The secondary structure of a protein refers to the folds and coils that are formed by hydrogen bonding between the slightly charged atoms of the polypeptide backbone. The primary structure is the sequence of amino acids, similar to the letters in a long word. The tertiary structure is the overall shape of the molecule that results from the interactions between the side chains that are linked to the polypeptide backbone. The quaternary structure is the complete protein structure that occurs when a protein is made up of two or more polypeptide chains.

23. C: In the Linnean system, organisms are classified as follows, moving from comprehensive and specific similarities to fewer and more general similarities: species, genus, family, order, class, phylum, kingdom, and domain. A popular mnemonic device to remember the Linnean system is "Dear King Philip came over for good soup."

24. A: All the other answer choices are functions of lipids. *B* is true because steroid hormones are lipid based. Long-term energy is one of the most important functions of lipids, so *C* is true. *D* is also true because the cell membrane is not only composed of a lipid bilayer, but it also has cholesterol (another lipid) embedded within it to regulate membrane fluidity.

25. D: Ribosomes are the structures responsible for protein synthesis using amino acids delivered by tRNA molecules. They are numerous within the cell and can take up as much as 25% of the cell. Ribosomes are found free-floating in the cytoplasm and also attached to the rough endoplasmic reticulum, which resides alongside the nucleus. Ribosomes translate messenger RNA into chains of amino acids that become proteins. Ribosomes themselves are made of protein as well as rRNA. Choice *B* might be an attractive choice, since the Golgi is the site of protein maturation; however, it is not where proteins are synthesized. Choice *A* might be an attractive choice as well because DNA provides the instructions for proteins to be made, but DNA does not make the protein itself.

Chemistry

Scientific Notation, the Metric System, and Temperature Scales

Scientific Notation
Scientific notation is the conversion of extremely small or large numbers into a format that is easier to comprehend and manipulate. It changes the number into three separate parts: a mathematical sign (+/-), a digit term (known as a **significand**), and an exponential term.

Scientific notation = (+ or -) significand x exponential term

To put a number into scientific notation, one should use the following steps:

- Move the decimal point to after the first non-zero number to find the digit number.
- Count how many places the decimal point was moved in step 1.
- Determine if the exponent is positive or negative.
- Create an exponential term using the information from steps 2 and 3.
- Combine the digit term and exponential term to get scientific notation.

For example, to put 0.0000098 into scientific notation, the decimal should be moved so that it lies between the last two numbers: 000009.8. This creates the digit number:

9.8

Next, the number of places that the decimal point moved is determined; to get between the 9 and the 8, the decimal was moved six places to the right. It may be helpful to remember that a decimal moved to the right creates a negative exponent, and a decimal moved to the left creates a positive exponent. Because the decimal was moved six places to the right, the exponent is negative.

Now, the exponential term can be created by using the base 10 (this is *always* the base in scientific notation) and the number of places moved as the exponent, in this case:

$$10^{-6}$$

Finally, the digit term and the exponential term can be combined as a product. Therefore, the scientific notation for the number 0.0000098 is:

$$9.8 \times 10^{-6}$$

Standard vs. Metric Systems
The measuring system used today in the United States developed from the British units of measurement during colonial times. The most typically used units in this customary system are those used to measure weight, liquid volume, and length, whose common units are found below. In the customary system, the basic unit for measuring weight is the ounce (oz); there are 16 ounces (oz) in 1 pound (lb) and 2000 pounds in 1 ton. The basic unit for measuring liquid volume is the ounce (oz); 1 ounce is equal to 2 tablespoons (tbsp) or 6 teaspoons (tsp), and there are 8 ounces in 1 cup, 2 cups in 1 pint (pt), 2 pints in 1 quart (qt), and 4 quarts in 1 gallon (gal). For measurements of length, the inch (in) is the base unit; 12 inches make up 1 foot (ft), 3 feet make up 1 yard (yd), and 5280 feet make up 1 mile (mi). However, as

there are only a set number of units in the customary system, with extremely large or extremely small amounts of material, the numbers can become awkward and difficult to compare.

Common Customary Measurements		
Length	Weight	Capacity
1 foot = 12 inches	1 pound = 16 ounces	1 cup = 8 fluid ounces
1 yard = 3 feet	1 ton = 2,000 pounds	1 pint = 2 cups
1 yard = 36 inches		1 quart = 2 pints
1 mile = 1,760 yards		1 quart = 4 cups
1 mile = 5,280 feet		1 gallon = 4 quarts
		1 gallon = 16 cups

Aside from the United States, most countries in the world have adopted the **metric system** embodied in the International System of Units (SI). The three main SI base units used in the metric system are the meter (m), the gram (g), and the liter (L); meters measure length, grams measure mass, and liters measure volume. These are known as the **basic units of measure.**

These three units can use different **prefixes**, which indicate larger or smaller versions of the unit by powers of ten. This can be thought of as making a new unit which is sized by multiplying the original unit in size by a factor.

These prefixes and associated factors are:

Metric Prefixes			
Prefix	Symbol	Multiplier	Exponential
kilo	k	1,000	10^3
hecto	h	100	10^2
deca	da	10	10^1
no prefix		1	10^0
deci	d	0.1	10^{-1}
centi	c	0.01	10^{-2}
milli	m	0.001	10^{-3}

The correct prefix is then attached to the base. Some examples:

1 milliliter equals .001 liters.

1 kilogram equals 1,000 grams.

Some units of measure are represented as square or cubic units depending on the solution. For example, perimeter is measured in units, area is measured in square units, and volume is measured in cubic units.

Also be sure to use the most appropriate unit for the thing being measured. A building's height might be measured in feet or meters while the length of a nail might be measured in inches or centimeters. Additionally, for SI units, the prefix should be chosen to provide the most succinct available value. For example, the mass of a bag of fruit would likely be measured in kilograms rather than grams or milligrams, and the length of a bacteria cell would likely be measured in micrometers rather than centimeters or kilometers.

Temperature Scales

There are three main temperature scales used in science. The scale most often used in the United States is the **Fahrenheit** scale. This scale is based on the measurement of water freezing at 32⁰ F and water boiling at 212⁰ F. The **Celsius** scale uses 0⁰ C as the temperature for water freezing and 100⁰ C for water boiling. The Celsius scale is the most widely used in the scientific community. The accepted measurement by the International System of Units (from the French *Système international d'unités*), or SI, for temperature is the **Kelvin** scale. This is the scale employed in thermodynamics, since its zero is the basis for *absolute zero*, or the unattainable temperature, when matter no longer exhibits degradation.

The conversions between the temperature scales are as follows:

⁰Fahrenheit to ⁰Celsius: $^0C = \frac{5}{9}(^0F - 32)$

⁰Celsius to ⁰Fahrenheit: $^0F = \frac{9}{5}(^0C) + 32$

⁰Celsius to Kelvin: $K = {}^0C + 273.15$

Accuracy and Precision

For a hypothesis to be proven true or false, all experiments are subject to multiple trials in order to verify accuracy and precision. A measurement is **accurate** if the observed value is close to the "true value." For example, if someone measured the pH of water at 6.9, this measurement would be considered accurate (the pH of water is 7). On the other hand, a measurement is **precise** if the measurements are consistent—that is, if they are reproducible. If someone had a series of values for a pH of water that were 6.9, 7.0, 7.2, and 7.3, their measurements would not be precise. However, if all measured values were 6.9, or the average of these values was 6.9 with a small range, then their measurements would be precise. Measurements can fall into the following categories:

- Both accurate and precise
- Accurate but not precise
- Precise but not accurate
- Neither accurate nor precise

Atomic Structure and the Periodic Table

Atomic Structure

The structure of an atom has two major components: the atomic nucleus and the atomic shells (also known as **orbits**). The **nucleus** is found in the center of an atom. The three major subatomic particles are protons, neutrons, and electrons and are found in the atomic nucleus and shells.

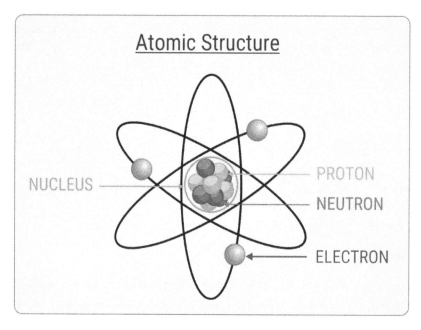

Protons are found in the atomic nucleus and are positively charged particles. The addition or removal of protons from an atom's nucleus creates an entirely different element. **Neutrons** are also found in the atomic nucleus and are neutral particles, meaning they have no net electrical charge. The addition or removal of neutrons from an atom's nucleus does not create a different element but instead creates a lighter or heavier form of that element called an isotope. **Electrons** are found orbiting in the atomic shells around the nucleus and are negatively charged particles. A proton or a neutron has nearly 2,000 times the mass of an electron.

Electrons orbit the nucleus in **atomic shells,** or **electron clouds**. For example, the first atomic shell can accommodate two electrons, the second atomic shell can hold a maximum of eight electrons, and the third atomic shell can house a maximum of eight electrons. The negatively charged electrons orbiting the nucleus are attracted to the positively charged protons in the nucleus via electromagnetic force. The attraction of opposite electrical charges gives rise to chemical bonds, which refers to the ways atoms are attached to each other.

The **atomic number** of an atom is determined by the number of protons within the nucleus. When a substance is composed of atoms that all have the same atomic number, it is called an **element**. Elements are arranged by atomic number and grouped by properties in the **Periodic table**.

An atom's **mass number** is determined by the sum of the total number of protons and neutrons in the atom. Most nuclei have a net neutral charge, and all atoms of one type have the same atomic number. However, there are some atoms of the same type that have a different mass number, due to an imbalance of neutrons. These are called **isotopes**. In isotopes, the atomic number, which is determined by the number of protons, is the same, but the mass number, which is determined by adding the protons and neutrons, is different due to the irregular number of neutrons.

An atom can gain a charge by having greater or fewer electrons than protons, and any atom with a charge is referred to as an **ion**. If an ion has more electrons than protons, it has a negative charge and is an **anion**. If an atom has fewer electrons than protons, it has a positive charge and is a **cation**.

Chemical Bonding
Chemical bonding typically results in the formation of a new substance, called a **compound**. Only the electrons in the outermost atomic shell are able to form chemical bonds. These electrons are known as **valence electrons**, and they are what determines the chemical properties of an atom.

Chemical bonding occurs between two or more atoms that are joined together. There are three types of chemical bonds: ionic, covalent, and metallic. The characteristics of the different bonds are determined by how electrons behave in a compound. **Lewis structures** were developed to help visualize the electrons in molecules; they are a method of writing a compound structure formula and including its electron composition. A Lewis symbol for an element consists of the element symbol and a dot for each valence electron. The dots are located on all four sides of the symbol, with a maximum of two dots per side, and eight dots, or electrons, total. The octet rule states that atoms tend to gain, lose, or share electrons until they have a total of eight valence electrons.

Ionic bonds are formed from the electrostatic attractions between oppositely charged atoms. They result from the transfer of electrons from a metal on the left side of the periodic table to a nonmetal on the right side. The metallic substance often has low ionization energy and will transfer an electron easily to the nonmetal, which has a high electron affinity. An example of this is the compound NaCl, which is sodium chloride or table salt, where the Na atom transfers an electron to the Cl atom. Due to strong bonding, ionic compounds have several distinct characteristics. They have high melting and boiling points and are brittle and crystalline. They are arranged in rigid, well-defined structures, which allow them to break apart along smooth, flat surfaces. The formation of ionic bonds is a reaction that is exothermic. In the opposite scenario, the energy it takes to break up a one mole quantity of an ionic compound is referred to as lattice energy, which is generally endothermic. The Lewis structure for NaCl is written as follows:

$$Na\cdot \ + \ :\ddot{Cl}\cdot \ \longrightarrow \ Na^+ \ +:\ddot{\underset{..}{Cl}}:$$

Covalent bonds are formed when two atoms share electrons, instead of transferring them as in ionic compounds. The atoms in covalent compounds have a balance of attraction and repulsion between their protons and electrons, which keeps them bonded together. Two atoms can be joined by single, double, or even triple covalent bonds. As the number of electrons that are shared increases, the length of the bond decreases. Covalent substances have low melting and boiling points and are poor conductors of heat and electricity.

The Lewis structure for Cl_2 is written as follows:

Lewis structure Cl_2

$$:\ddot{Cl}\cdot \ + \ \cdot\ddot{Cl}: \ \longrightarrow \ :\ddot{Cl}:\ddot{Cl}:$$

Metallic bonds are formed by electrons that move freely through metal. They are the product of the force of attraction between electrons and metal ions. The electrons are shared by many metal cations and act like glue that holds the metallic substance together, similar to the attraction between oppositely-charged atoms in ionic substances, except the electrons are more fluid and float around the bonded metals and form a sea of electrons. Metallic compounds have characteristic properties that include strength, conduction of heat and electricity, and malleability. They can conduct electricity by passing energy through the freely moving electrons, creating a **current**. These compounds also have high melting and boiling points. Lewis structures are not common for metallic structures because of the free-roaming ability of the electrons.

Periodic Table
The periodic table catalogues all of the elements known to man, currently 118. It is one of the most important references in the science of chemistry. Information that can be gathered from the periodic table includes the element's atomic number, atomic mass, and chemical symbol. The first periodic table was rendered by Mendeleev in the mid-1800s and was ordered according to increasing atomic mass. The modern periodic table is arranged in order of increasing atomic number. It is also arranged in horizontal rows known as **periods,** and vertical columns known as **families,** or **groups**. The periodic table contains seven periods and eighteen families. Elements in the periodic table can also be classified into three major groups: metals, metalloids, and nonmetals. **Metals** are concentrated on the left side of the periodic table, while **nonmetals** are found on the right side. **Metalloids** occupy the area between the metals and nonmetals.

Due to the fact the periodic table is ordered by increasing atomic number, the electron configurations of the elements show periodicity. As the atomic number increases, electrons gradually fill the shells of an atom. In general, the start of a new period corresponds to the first time an electron inhabits a new shell.

Periodic Table of the Elements

Other trends in the properties of elements in the periodic table are:

Atomic radius: One-half the distance between the nuclei of atoms of the same element.

Electronegativity: A measurement of the willingness of an atom to form a chemical bond.

Ionization energy: The amount of energy needed to remove an electron from a gas or ion.

Electron affinity: The ability of an atom to accept an electron.

Trends in the Periodic Table

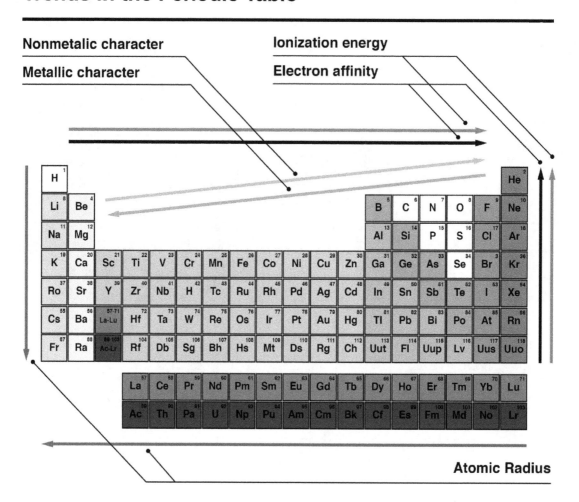

Nonmetalic character

Metallic character

Ionization energy

Electron affinity

Atomic Radius

Chemical Equations

Chemical reactions are represented by **chemical equations**. The equations help to explain how the molecules change during the reaction. For example, when hydrogen gas (H_2) combines with oxygen gas (O_2), two molecules of water are formed. The equation is written as follows, where the "+" sign means *reacts with* and the "→" means *produces*:

$$2\,H_2 + O_2 \rightarrow 2\,H_2O$$

Two hydrogen molecules react with an oxygen molecule to produce two water molecules. In all chemical equations, the quantity of each element on the reactant side of the equation should equal the quantity of the same element on the product side of the equation due to the law of conservation of matter. If this is true, the equation is described as balanced. To figure out how many of each element there is on each side of the equation, the coefficient of the element should be multiplied by the subscript next to the element. Coefficients and subscripts are noted for quantities larger than one. The **coefficient** is the number located directly to the left of the element. The **subscript** is the small-sized number directly to the right of the element. In the equation above, on the left side, the coefficient of the hydrogen is two and the subscript is also two, which makes a total of four hydrogen atoms. Using the same method, there are two oxygen atoms. On the right side, the coefficient two is multiplied by the subscript in each element of the water molecule, making four hydrogen atoms and two oxygen atoms. This equation is balanced because there are four hydrogen atoms and two oxygen atoms on each side. The states of the reactants and products can also be written in the equation: gas (g), liquid (l), solid (s), and dissolved in water (aq). If they are included, they are noted in parentheses on the right side of each molecule in the equation.

Reaction Rates, Equilibrium, and Reversibility

Chemical reactions are conveyed using chemical equations. Chemical equations must be balanced with equivalent numbers of atoms for each type of element on each side of the equation. Antoine Lavoisier, a French chemist, was the first to propose the **Law of Conservation of Mass** for the purpose of balancing a chemical equation. The law states, "Matter is neither created nor destroyed during a chemical reaction."

The **reactants** are located on the left side of the arrow, while the **products** are located on the right side of the arrow. Coefficients are the numbers in front of the chemical formulas. Subscripts are the numbers to the lower right of chemical symbols in a formula. To tally atoms, one should multiply the formula's coefficient by the subscript of each chemical symbol. For example, the chemical equation $2\,H_2 + O_2 \rightarrow 2\,H_2O$ is balanced. For H, the coefficient of 2 multiplied by the subscript 2 = 4 hydrogen atoms. For O, the coefficient of 1 multiplied by the subscript 2 = 2 oxygen atoms. Coefficients and subscripts of 1 are understood and never written.

States of Matter and Factors that Affect Phase Changes

Matter is most commonly found in three distinct states or phases: solid, liquid, and gas. A solid has a distinct shape and a defined volume. A liquid has a more loosely defined shape and a definite volume, while a gas has no definite shape or volume. The *Kinetic Theory of Matter* states that matter is composed of a large number of small particles (specifically, atoms and molecules) that are in constant motion. The distance between the separations in these particles determines the state of the matter: solid, liquid, or gas. In gases, the particles have a large separation and no attractive forces. In liquids, there is moderate separation between particles and some attractive forces to form a loose shape. Solids have almost no separation between their particles, causing a defined and set shape. The constant movement of particles causes them to bump into each other, thus allowing the particles to transfer energy between each other. This bumping and transferring of energy helps explain the transfer of heat and the relationship between pressure, volume, and temperature.

The *Ideal Gas Law* states that pressure, volume, and temperature are all related through the equation: $PV = nRT$, where P is pressure, V is volume, n is the amount of the substance in moles, R is the gas constant, and T is temperature.

Through this relationship, volume and pressure are both proportional to temperature, but pressure is inversely proportional to volume. Therefore, if the equation is balanced, and the volume decreases in the system, pressure needs to proportionately increase to keep both sides of the equation balanced. In contrast, if the equation is unbalanced and the pressure increases, then the temperature would also increase, since pressure and temperature are directly proportional.

When pressure, temperature, or volume change in matter, a change in state can occur. Changes in state include solid to liquid (melting), liquid to gas (evaporation), solid to gas (sublimation), gas to solid (deposition), gas to liquid (condensation), and liquid to solid (freezing). There is one other state of matter called *plasma*, which is seen in lightning, television screens, and neon lights. Plasma is most commonly converted from the gas state at extremely high temperatures.

The amount of energy needed to change matter from one state to another is labeled by the terms for phase changes. For example, the temperature needed to supply enough energy for matter to change from a liquid to a gas is called the *heat of vaporization*. When heat is added to matter in order to cause a change in state, there will be an increase in temperature until the matter is about to change its state. During its transition, all of the added heat is used by the matter to change its state, so there is no increase in temperature. Once the transition is complete, then the added heat will again yield an increase in temperature.

Reaction Rates

The rate of a reaction is the measure of the change in concentration of the reactants or products over a certain period of time. Many factors affect how fast or slow a reaction occurs, such as concentration, pressure, or temperature. As the concentration of a reactant increases, the rate of the reaction also increases, because the frequency of collisions between elements increases. High-pressure situations for reactants that are gases cause the gas to compress and increase the frequency of gas molecule collisions, similar to solutions with higher concentrations. Reactions rates are then increased with the higher frequency of gas molecule collisions. Higher temperatures usually increase the rate of the reaction, adding more energy to the system with heat and increasing the frequency of molecular collisions.

Equilibrium

Equilibrium is described as the state of a system when no net changes occur. Chemical equilibrium occurs when opposing reactions occur at equal rates. In other words, the rate of reactants forming products is equal to the rate of the products breaking down into the reactants—the concentration of reactants and products in the system doesn't change. This happens in **reversible chemical reactions** as opposed to irreversible chemical reactions. In **irreversible chemical reactions**, the products cannot be changed back to reactants. Although the concentrations are not changing in equilibrium, the forward and reverse reactions are likely still occurring. This type of equilibrium is called a **dynamic equilibrium**. In situations where all reactions have ceased, a **static equilibrium** is reached. Chemical equilibriums are also described as homogeneous or heterogeneous. **Homogeneous equilibrium** involves substances that are all in the same phase, while **heterogeneous equilibrium** means the substances are in different phases when equilibrium is reached.

When a reaction reaches equilibrium, the conditions of the equilibrium are described by the following equation, based on the chemical equation $aA + bB \leftrightarrow cC + dD$:

Catalysts are substances that accelerate the speed of a chemical reaction. A catalyst remains unchanged throughout the course of a chemical reaction. In most cases, only small amounts of a catalyst are needed. Catalysts increase the rate of a chemical reaction by providing an alternate path requiring less activation energy. Activation energy refers to the amount of energy required for the initiation of a chemical reaction.

Catalysts can be homogeneous or heterogeneous. Catalysts in the same phase of matter as its reactants are homogeneous, while catalysts in a different phase than reactants are heterogeneous. It is important to remember catalysts are selective. They don't accelerate the speed of all chemical reactions, but catalysts do accelerate specific chemical reactions.

Solutions and Solution Concentrations

A homogeneous mixture, also called a **solution,** has uniform properties throughout a given sample. An example of a homogeneous solution is salt (the **solute,** or what is being dissolved) fully dissolved in warm water (the **solvent,** the material dissolving the solute). In this example, salt is the **solute,** or the material being dissolved, and water is the **solvent,** or the material dissolving the solute. In this case, any number of samples taken from the parent solution would be identical.

One **mole** is the amount of matter contained in 6.02×10^{23} of any object, such as atoms, ions, or molecules. It is a useful unit of measure for items in large quantities. This number is also known as **Avogadro's number**. One mole of ^{12}C atoms is equivalent to 6.02×10^{23} ^{12}C atoms. Avogadro's number is often written as an inverse mole, or as $6.02 \times 10^{23}/mol$.

Molarity is the concentration of a solution. It is based on the number of moles of solute in one liter of solution and is written as the capital letter M. A 1.0 molar solution, or 1.0 M solution, has one mole of solute per liter of solution. The molarity of a solution can be determined by calculating the number of moles of the solute and dividing it by the volume of the solution in liters. The resulting number is the mol/L or M for molarity of the solution. Alternatively, **percent concentration** can be written as parts of solute per 100 parts of solvent.

Chemical Reactions

Chemical reactions are characterized by a chemical change in which the starting substances, or reactants, differ from the substances formed, or products. Chemical reactions may involve a change in color, the production of gas, the formation of a precipitate, or changes in heat content. The following are the five basic types of chemical reactions:

- **Decomposition Reactions:** A compound is broken down into smaller elements. For example, $2H_2O \rightarrow 2H_2 + O_2$. This is read as, "2 molecules of water decompose into 2 molecules of hydrogen and 1 molecule of oxygen."

- **Synthesis Reactions:** Two or more elements or compounds are joined together. For example, $2H_2 + O_2 \rightarrow 2H_2O$. This is read as, "2 molecules of hydrogen react with 1 molecule of oxygen to produce 2 molecules of water."

- **Single Displacement Reactions:** A single element or ion takes the place of another element in a compound. It is also known as a substitution reaction. For example, $Zn + 2 HCl \rightarrow ZnCl_2 + H_2$. This is read as, "zinc reacts with 2 molecules of hydrochloric acid to produce one molecule of zinc chloride and one molecule of hydrogen." In other words, zinc replaces the hydrogen in hydrochloric acid.

- **Double Displacement Reactions:** Two elements or ions exchange a single element to form two different compounds, resulting in different combinations of cations and anions in the final compounds. It is also known as a metathesis reaction. For example, $H_2SO_4 + 2 NaOH \rightarrow Na_2 SO_4 + 2 H_2O$

    - Special types of double displacement reactions include:

        - **Oxidation-Reduction (or Redox) Reactions:** Elements undergo a change in oxidation number. For example, $2 S_2O_3^{2-}$ (aq) $+ I_2$ (aq) $\rightarrow S_4O_6^{2-}$ (aq) $+ 2 I^-$ (aq).

- **Acid-Base Reactions:** Involves a reaction between an acid and a base, which produces a salt and water. For example, $HBr + NaOH \rightarrow NaBr + H_2O$.

- **Combustion Reactions:** A hydrocarbon (a compound composed of only hydrogen and carbon) reacts with oxygen (O_2) to form carbon dioxide (CO_2) and water (H_2O). For example, $CH_4 + 2O_2 \rightarrow CO_2 + 2H_2O$.

Stoichiometry

Stoichiometry investigates the quantities of chemicals that are consumed and produced in chemical reactions. Chemical equations are made up of reactants and products; stoichiometry helps elucidate how the changes from reactants to products occur, as well as how to ensure the equation is balanced.

Chemical reactions are limited by the amount of starting material, or reactants, available to drive the process forward. The reactant that has the smallest amount of substance is called the limiting reactant. The **limiting reactant** is completely consumed by the end of the reaction. The other reactants are called **excess reactants**. For example, gasoline is used in a combustion reaction to make a car move and is the limiting reactant of the reaction. If the gasoline runs out, the combustion reaction can no longer take place, and the car stops.

The quantity of product that should be produced after using up all of the limiting reactant can be calculated and is called the **theoretical yield of the reaction**. Since the reactants do not always act as they should, the actual amount of resulting product is called the **actual yield**. The actual yield is divided by the theoretical yield and then multiplied by 100 to find the **percent yield** for the reaction.

Solution stoichiometry deals with quantities of solutes in chemical reactions that occur in solutions. The quantity of a solute in a solution can be calculated by multiplying the molarity of the solution by the volume. Similar to chemical equations involving simple elements, the number of moles of the elements that make up the solute should be equivalent on both sides of the equation.

When the concentration of a particular solute in a solution is unknown, a **titration** is used to determine that concentration. In a titration, the solution with the unknown solute is combined with a standard solution, which is a solution with a known solute concentration. The point at which the unknown solute has completely reacted with the known solute is called the **equivalence point**. Using the known information about the standard solution, including the concentration and volume, and the volume of the unknown solution, the concentration of the unknown solute is determined in a balanced equation. For example, in the case of combining acids and bases, the equivalence point is reached when the resulting solution is neutral. HCl, an acid, combines with NaOH, a base, to form water, which is neutral, and a solution of Cl^- ions and Na^+ ions. Before the equivalence point, there are an unequal number of cations and anions and the solution is not neutral.

Oxidation and Reduction

Oxidation and reduction reactions, also known as **redox reactions**, are those in which electrons are transferred from one element to another. Batteries and fuel cells are two energy-related technologies that utilize these reactions. When an atom, ion, or molecule loses its electrons and becomes more positively charged, it is described as being oxidized. When a substance gains electrons and becomes more negatively charged, it is reduced. In chemical reactions, if one element or molecule is oxidized, another must be reduced for the equation to be balanced. Although the transfer of electrons is obvious in some reactions where ions are formed, redox reactions also include those in which electrons are transferred but the products remain neutral.

Keep track of oxidation states or oxidation numbers to ensure the chemical equation is balanced. **Oxidation numbers** are assigned to each atom in a neutral substance or ion. For ions made up of a single atom, the oxidation number is equal to the charge of the ion. For atoms in their original elemental form, the oxidation number is always zero. Each hydrogen atom in an H_2 molecule, for example, has an oxidation number of zero. The sum of the oxidation numbers in a molecule should be equal to the overall charge of the molecule. If the molecule is a positively charged ion, the sum of the oxidation number should be equal to overall positive charge of the molecule. In ionic compounds that have a cation and anion joined, the sum of the oxidation numbers should equal zero.

All chemical equations must have the same number of elements on each side of the equation to be balanced. Redox reactions have an extra step of counting the electrons on both sides of the equation to be balanced. Separating redox reactions into oxidation reactions and reduction reactions is a simple way to account for all of the electrons involved. The individual equations are known as **half-reactions**. The number of electrons lost in the oxidation reaction must be equal to the number of electrons gained in the reduction reaction for the redox reaction to be balanced.

The oxidation of tin (Sn) by iron (Fe) can be balanced by the following half-reactions:

Oxidation: $Sn^{2+} \rightarrow Sn^{4+} + 2e^-$

Reduction: $2Fe^{3+} + 2e^- \rightarrow 2Fe^{2+}$

Complete redox reaction: $Sn^{2+} + 2Fe^{3+} \rightarrow Sn^{4+} + 2Fe^{2+}$

Acids and Bases

Acids and bases are defined in many different ways. An **acid** can be described as a substance that increases the concentration of H^+ ions when it is dissolved in water, as a proton donor in a chemical equation, or as an electron-pair acceptor. A **base** can be a substance that increases the concentration of OH^- ions when it is dissolved in water, accepts a proton in a chemical reaction, or is an electron-pair donor.

pH refers to the power or potential of hydrogen atoms and is used as a scale for a substance's acidity. In chemistry, pH represents the hydrogen ion concentration (written as $[H^+]$) in an aqueous, or watery, solution. The hydrogen ion concentration, $[H^+]$, is measured in moles of H^+ per liter of solution.

The pH scale is a logarithmic scale used to quantify how acidic or basic a substance is. pH is the negative logarithm of the hydrogen ion concentration: $pH = -\log[H^+]$. A one-unit change in pH correlates with a ten-fold change in hydrogen ion concentration. The pH scale typically ranges from zero to 14, although it is possible to have pHs outside of this range. Pure water has a pH of 7, which is considered **neutral**. pH values less than 7 are considered **acidic**, while pH values greater than 7 are considered **basic**, or **alkaline**.

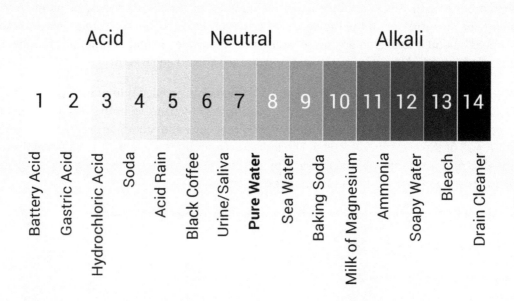

Generally speaking, an acid is a substance capable of donating hydrogen ions, while a base is a substance capable of accepting hydrogen ions. A **buffer** is a molecule that can act as either a hydrogen ion donor or acceptor. Buffers are crucial in the blood and body fluids, and prevent the body's pH from fluctuating into dangerous territory. pH can be measured using a pH meter, test paper, or indicator sticks.

Water can act as either an acid or a base. When mixed with an acid, water can accept a proton and become an H_3O^+ ion. When mixed with a base, water can donate a proton and become an OH^- ion. Sometimes water molecules donate and accept protons from each other; this process is called **autoionization**. The chemical equation is written as follows: $H_2O + H_2O \rightarrow OH^- + H_3O^+$.

Acids and bases are characterized as strong, weak, or somewhere in between. Strong acids and bases completely or almost completely ionize in aqueous solution. The chemical reaction is driven completely forward, to the right side of the equation, where the acidic or basic ions are formed. Weak acids and bases do not completely disassociate in aqueous solution. They only partially ionize and the solution becomes a mixture of the acid or base, water, and the acidic or basic ions. Strong acids are complemented by weak bases, and vice versa. A **conjugate acid** is an ion that forms when its base pair gains a proton. For example, the conjugate acid NH_4^+ is formed from the base NH_3. The **conjugate base** that pairs with an acid is the ion that is formed when an acid loses a proton. NO_2^- is the conjugate base of the acid HNO_2.

Nuclear Chemistry

Nuclear chemistry is the study of reactions in which the nuclei of atoms are transformed and their identities are changed. These reactions can involve large changes in energy—much larger than the energy changes that occur when chemical bonds between atoms are made or broken. Nuclear chemistry is also used to create electricity.

Nuclear reactions are described by nuclear equations, which have different notations than regular chemical equations. Nuclear equations are written as follows, with the top number being the **atomic mass** and the bottom number being the atomic number for each element:

$$^{238}_{92}U \rightarrow\ ^{234}_{90}Th + ^{4}_{2}He$$

The equation describes the spontaneous decomposition of uranium into thorium and helium via alpha decay. When this happens, the process is referred to as nuclear decay. Similar to chemical equations, nuclear equations must be balanced on each side; the sum of the mass numbers and the sum of the atomic numbers should be equal on both sides of the equation.

In some cases, the nucleus of an atom is unstable and constantly emits particles due to this instability. These atoms are described as radioactive and the isotopes are referred to as **radioisotopes.** There are three types of radioactive decay that occur most frequently: alpha (α), beta (β), and gamma (γ). **Alpha radiation** is emitted when a nucleus releases a stream of alpha particles, which are helium-4 nuclei. **Beta radiation** occurs when a stream of high-speed electrons is emitted by an unstable nucleus. The beta particles are often noted as β^-. **Gamma radiation** occurs when the nucleus emits high-energy photons. In gamma radiation, the atomic number and the mass remain the same for the unstable nucleus. This type of radiation represents a rearrangement of an unstable nucleus into a more stable one and often accompanies other types of radioactive emission. **Radioactive decay** is often described in terms of its half-life, which is the time that it takes for half of the radioactive substance to react. For example, the radioisotope strontium-90 has a half-life of 28.8 years. If there are 10 grams of strontium-90 to start with, after 28.8 years, there would be 5 grams left.

There are two distinct types of nuclear reactions: fission and fusion reactions. Both involve a large energy release. In **fission** reactions, a large atom is split into two or more smaller atoms. The nucleus absorbs slow-moving neutrons, resulting in a larger nucleus that is unstable. The unstable nucleus then undergoes fission. Nuclear power plants depend on nuclear fission reactions for energy. **Fusion** reactions involve the combination of two or more lighter atoms into a larger atom. Fusion reactions do not occur in Earth's nature due to the extreme temperature and pressure conditions required to make them happen. Fusion products are generally not radioactive. Fusion reactions are responsible for the energy that is created by the Sun.

Biochemistry

Biochemistry deals with the chemistry of organisms. There are four classes of macromolecules that allow organisms to exist: carbohydrates, lipids, proteins, and nucleic acids. Carbon is the backbone of these organic molecules because of its ability to form up to four covalent bonds. Carbon (C), hydrogen

(H), oxygen (O), nitrogen (N), sulfur (S), and phosphorus (P) are the most prevalent elements in these biological molecules. The following chart gives an overview of each organic molecule.

Organic Molecule	Example	Monomer (smallest repeating unit)	Structure	Function
Carbohydrate	• Sugar • Cellulose	Monosaccharide	 Glucose　　Fructose　　Galactose	• Energy • Structure
Protein	• Actin • Insulin	Amino Acid		• Structure • Support • Some hormones
Lipid	• Fat • Oil	Technically none because the glycerol and fatty acids are not repeating.	 Glycerol　　　　Triglyceride-Saturated	• Long-term energy • Steroid Hormones • Cell membranes
Nucleic Acid	• DNA • RNA	Nucleotide		• Genetic code • Makes Protein

Carbohydrates

Carbohydrates are usually sweet, ring-like sugar molecules that are built from carbon (carbo-) and oxygen & hydrogen (-hydrates, meaning water). They can exist as one-ring **monosaccharides,** like glucose, fructose, and galactose, or as two-ring **disaccharides**, like lactose, maltose, and sucrose. These simple sugars can be easily broken down and used via glycolysis to provide a source of quick energy. **Polysaccharides** are repeating chains of monosaccharide rings. They are more complex carbohydrates, and there are several types. For example:

- Plants store energy in the form of **starch**.
- Animals store energy in the form of **glycogen**. Vertebrates store glycogen in the liver and muscles.
- **Cellulose** is the chief structural component of plant cell walls.
- **Chitin** is the chief structural component of fungi cell walls and the exoskeletons of arthropods.

Glycolysis is an essential metabolic pathway that converts glucose to pyruvate and allows for cellular respiration to occur. It does not require oxygen to be present. Glucose is a common molecule used for energy production in cells. During glycolysis, two three-carbon sugars are generated from the splitting of a glucose molecule. These smaller sugars are then converted into pyruvate molecules via oxidation and atom rearrangement. Glycolysis requires two ATP molecules to drive the process forward, but the end product of the process has four ATP molecules, for a net production of two ATP molecules. Also, two reduced nicotinamide adenine dinucleotide (NADH) molecules are created from when the electron carrier oxidized nicotinamide adenine dinucleotide (NAD+) peels off two electrons and a hydrogen atom.

Proteins

Proteins are composed of chains of amino acids. There are several different kinds.

- **Enzymes** catalyze chemical reactions in the body.

- **Storage proteins** like albumin in eggs are important for development.

- **Hormonal proteins** are responsible for initiating signal transduction cascades that regulate gene expression.

- **Motor proteins** like actin and myosin are responsible for movement.

- **Immune proteins** like antibodies and antigens are important for fighting disease.

- **Transport proteins** like channel proteins and protein pumps move molecules.

- **Receptor proteins** receive chemical messages like neurotransmitters.

- **Marker proteins** serve as a cell's identification or fingerprint that distinguishes between cells of different types and sources.

- **Structural proteins** like keratin are important for things like spider webs, hair, and feathers.

All proteins are made from a combination of 20 amino acids. The varying amino acids are linked by **peptide bonds** and form the primary structure of the **polypeptide**, or chain of amino acids. The primary structure is just the string of amino acids. It is the secondary, tertiary, and quaternary structure that determines protein shape and function. The secondary structure can be beta sheets or alpha helices formed by hydrogen bonding between the polar regions of the polypeptide backbone. Tertiary structure results from the interactions between the side chains. Quaternary structure is the overall protein structure that occurs when subunits merge, take the correct shape, and become functional.

The process of breaking down proteins to produce glucose is **gluconeogenesis.**

Lipids

Lipids are mostly nonpolar, hydrophobic molecules that are not soluble in water. **Triglycerides** are a type of lipid with a glycerol backbone attached to three long fatty acid chains.

Phospholipids are also composed of glycerol except they have two fatty acid tails. The third tail is replaced with a hydrophilic phosphate group. The amphipathic nature of this molecule results in a lipid bilayer where the "water-loving" hydrophilic heads face the extracellular matrix and cytoplasm and the "water-hating" hydrophobic tails face each other on the inside.

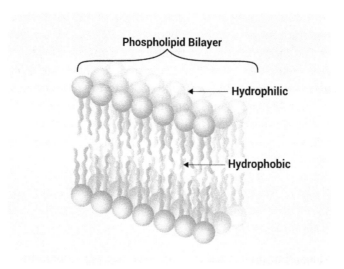

Steroids are another type of lipid. Cholesterol is a steroid that embeds itself in animal cell membranes and acts as a fluidity buffer. Steroid hormones such as testosterone and estrogen are responsible for transcriptional regulation in certain cells.

Nucleic acids

Nucleic acids are made of **nucleotides**. Nucleotides consist of a five-carbon sugar, a nitrogen-containing base, and a phosphate group. Deoxyribonucleic acid (DNA) exists as two nucleotide chains arranged in a double helix. Each **deoxyribose** sugar is connected to a nitrogen base and an electrically negative phosphate group. The nitrogen bases are adenine and guanine, the two-ringed purines, and cytosine and thymine, the one-ringed pyrimidines. The double helix is held together by weak hydrogen bonds that connect adenine to thymine and cytosine to guanine. Ribonucleic acid (RNA) has a slightly different structure. It is usually single-stranded, has a **ribose** sugar as opposed to deoxyribose, and contains uracil instead of thymine.

Practice Questions

1. Which of the following is a special property of water?
    a. Water easily flows through phospholipid bilayers.
    b. A water molecule's oxygen atom allows fish to breathe.
    c. Water is highly cohesive which explains its high melting point.
    d. Water can self-hydrolyze and decompose into hydrogen and oxygen.

2. What is the electrical charge of the nucleus?
    a. A nucleus always has a positive charge.
    b. A stable nucleus has a positive charge, but a radioactive nucleus may have no charge and instead be neutral.
    c. A nucleus always has no charge and is instead neutral.
    d. A stable nucleus has no charge and is instead neutral, but a radioactive nucleus may have a charge.

3. What is the temperature in Fahrenheit when it is 35°C outside?
    a. 67°F
    b. 95°F
    c. 63°F
    d. 75°F

4. How are a sodium atom and a sodium isotope different?
    a. The isotope has a different number of protons.
    b. The isotope has a different number of neutrons.
    c. The isotope has a different number of electrons.
    d. The isotope has a different atomic number.

5. Which statement is true about nonmetals?
    a. They form cations.
    b. They form covalent bonds.
    c. They are mostly absent from organic compounds.
    d. They are all diatomic.

6. What is the basic unit of matter?
    a. Elementary particle
    b. Atom
    c. Molecule
    d. Photon

7. Which particle is responsible for all chemical reactions?
    a. Electrons
    b. Neutrons
    c. Protons
    d. Orbitals

8. Which of these give atoms a negative charge?
    a. Electrons
    b. Neutrons
    c. Protons
    d. Orbital

9. How are similar chemical properties of elements grouped on the periodic table?
    a. In rows according to their total configuration of electrons
    b. In columns according to the electron configuration in their outer shells
    c. In rows according to the electron configuration in their outer shells
    d. In columns according to their total configurations of electrons

10. In a chemical equation, the reactants are on which side of the arrow?
    a. Right
    b. Left
    c. Neither right nor left
    d. Both right and left

11. What does the law of conservation of mass state?
    a. All matter is equally created.
    b. Matter changes but is not created.
    c. Matter can be changed, and new matter can be created
    d. Matter can be created, but not changed.

12. Which factors decrease solubility of solids?
    a. Heating
    b. Agitation
    c. Large Surface area
    d. Decreasing solvent

13. What information is used to calculate the quantity of solute in a solution?
    a. Molarity of the solution
    b. Equivalence point
    c. Limiting reactant
    d. Theoretical yield

14. How does adding salt to water affect its boiling point?
    a. It increases it.
    b. It has no effect.
    c. It decreases it.
    d. It prevents it from boiling.

15. What is the effect of pressure on a liquid solution?
    a. It decreases solubility.
    b. It increases solubility.
    c. It has little effect on solubility.
    d. It has the same effect as with a gaseous solution.

16. Nonpolar molecules must have what kind regions?
   a. Hydrophilic
   b. Hydrophobic
   c. Hydrolytic
   d. Hydrochloric

17. Which of these is a substance that increases the rate of a chemical reaction?
   a. Catalyst
   b. Brine
   c. Solvent
   d. Inhibitor

18. Which of the following are composed of chains of amino acids?
   a. Lipids
   b. Nucleic Acids
   c. Proteins
   d. Carbohydrates

19. What is the balance of the following combustion equation?

$$\_C_2H_{10} + \_O_2 \rightarrow \_H_2O + \_CO_2$$

   a. 1:5:5:2
   b. 1:9:5:2
   c. 2: 9:10:4
   d. 2:5:10:4

20. Which type of bonding results from transferring electrons between atoms?
   a. Ionic bonding
   b. Covalent bonding
   c. Hydrogen bonding
   d. Dipole interactions

21. Which substance is oxidized in the following reaction?

$$4Fe + 3O_2 \rightarrow 2Fe_2O_3$$

   a. Fe
   b. O
   c. O_2
   d. Fe_2O_3

22. Which statements are true regarding nuclear fission?
   I. Splitting of heavy nuclei
   II. Utilized in power plants
   III. Occurs on the sun
   a. I only
   b. II and III only
   c. I and II only
   d. III only

23. Which type of nuclear decay is occurring in the equation below?

$$U_{92}^{236} \rightarrow He_2^4 + Th_{90}^{232}$$

    a. Alpha
    b. Beta
    c. Gamma
    d. Delta

24. Which statement is true about the pH of a solution?
    a. A solution cannot have a pH less than 1.
    b. The more hydroxide ions there are in the solution, the higher the pH will be.
    c. If an acid has a pH of greater than -2, it is considered a weak acid.
    d. A solution with a pH of 2 has ten times the amount of hydronium ions than a solution with a pH of 1.

25. Which radioactive particle is the most penetrating and damaging and is used to treat cancer in radiation?
    a. Alpha
    b. Beta
    c. Gamma
    d. Delta

Answer Explanations

1. C: Water's polarity lends it to be extremely cohesive and adhesive; this cohesion keeps its atoms very close together. Because of this, it takes a large amount of energy to melt and boil its solid and liquid forms. Phospholipid bilayers are made of nonpolar lipids and water, a polar liquid, cannot flow through it. Cell membranes use proteins called aquaporins to solve this issue and let water flow in and out. Fish breathe by capturing dissolved oxygen through their gills. Water can self-ionize, wherein it decomposes into a hydrogen ion (H^+) and a hydroxide ion (OH^-), but it cannot self-hydrolyze.

2. A: The neutrons and protons make up the nucleus of the atom. The nucleus is positively charged due to the presence of the protons. The negatively charged electrons are attracted to the positively charged nucleus by the electrostatic or Coulomb force; however, the electrons are not contained in the nucleus. The positively charged protons create the positive charge in the nucleus, and the neutrons are electrically neutral, so they have no effect. Radioactivity does not directly have a bearing on the charge of the nucleus.

3. B: The conversion from Celsius to Fahrenheit is $°F = \frac{9}{5}(°C) + 32$. Substituting the value for °C gives $°F = \frac{9}{5}(35) + 32$ which yields 95°F. The other choices do not apply the formula correctly and completely.

4. B: Choices A and D both suggest a different number of protons, which would make a different element. It would no longer be a sodium atom if the proton number or atomic number were different, so those are both incorrect. An atom that has a different number of electrons is called an ion, so choice C is incorrect as well.

5. B: They form covalent bonds. If nonmetals form ionic bonds, they will fill their electron orbital (and become an anion) rather than lose electrons (and become a cation), due to their smaller atomic radius and higher electronegativity than metals. A is, therefore, incorrect. There are some nonmetals that are diatomic (hydrogen, oxygen, nitrogen, and halogens), but that is not true for all of them; thus, D is incorrect. Organic compounds are carbon-based due to carbon's ability to form four covalent bonds. In addition to carbon, organic compounds are also rich in hydrogen, phosphorous, nitrogen, oxygen, and sulfur, so C is incorrect as well.

6. B: The basic unit of matter is the atom. Each element is identified by a letter symbol for that element and an atomic number, which indicates the number of protons in that element. Atoms are the building block of each element and are comprised of a nucleus that contains protons (positive charge) and neutrons (no charge). Orbiting around the nucleus at varying distances are negatively-charged electrons. An electrically-neutral atom contains equal numbers of protons and electrons. Atomic mass is the combined mass of protons and neutrons in the nucleus. Electrons have such negligible mass that they are not considered in the atomic mass. Although the nucleus is compact, the electrons orbit in energy levels at great relative distances to it, making an atom mostly empty space.

7. A: Nuclear reactions involve the nucleus, and chemical reactions involve electron behavior alone. If electrons are transferred between atoms, they form ionic bonds. If they are shared between atoms, they form covalent bonds. Unequal sharing within a covalent bond results in intermolecular attractions, including hydrogen bonding. Metallic bonding involves a "sea of electrons," where they float around non-specifically, resulting in metal ductility and malleability, due to their glue-like effect of sticking neighboring atoms together. Their metallic bonding also contributes to electrical conductivity and low specific heats, due to electrons' quick response to charge and heat, given to their mobility. Their floating also results in metals' property of luster as light reflects off the mobile electrons. Electron movement in any type of bond is enhanced by photon and heat energy investments, increasing their likelihood to jump energy levels. Valence electron status is the ultimate contributor to electron behavior as it determines their likelihood to be transferred or shared.

8. A: Electrons give atoms their negative charge. Electron behavior determines their bonding, and bonding can either be covalent (electrons are shared) or ionic (electrons are transferred). The charge of an atom is determined by the electrons in its orbitals. Electrons give atoms their chemical and electromagnetic properties. Unequal numbers of protons and electrons lend either a positive or negative charge to the atom. Ions are atoms with a charge, either positive or negative.

9. B: On the periodic table, the elements are grouped in columns according to the configuration of electrons in their outer orbitals. The groupings on the periodic table give a broad view of trends in chemical properties for the elements. The outer electron shell (or orbital) is most important in determining the chemical properties of the element. The electrons in this orbital determine charge and bonding compatibility. The number of electron shells increases by row from top to bottom. The periodic table is organized with elements that have similar chemical behavior in the columns (groups or families).

10. B: In chemical equations, the reactants are on the left side of the arrow. The direction of the reaction is in the direction of the arrow, although sometimes reactions will be shown with arrows in both directions, meaning the reaction is reversible. The reactants are on the left, and the products of the reaction are on the right side of the arrow. Chemical equations indicate atomic and molecular bond formations, rearrangements, and dissolutions. The numbers in front of the elements are called coefficients, and they designate the number of moles of that element accounted for in the reaction. The subscript numbers tell how many atoms of that element are in the molecule, with the number "1" being understood. In H_2O, for example, there are two atoms of hydrogen bound to one atom of oxygen. The ionic charge of the element is shown in superscripts and can be either positive or negative.

11. B: The law of conservation of mass states that matter cannot be created or destroyed, but that it can change forms. This is important in balancing chemical equations on both sides of the arrow. Unbalanced equations will have an unequal number of atoms of each element on either side of the equation and violate the law.

12. D: Solids all increase solubility with choices A-C. Powdered hot chocolate is an example to consider. Heating (*A*) and stirring (*B*) make it dissolve faster. Regarding Choice *C*, powder is in chunks that collectively result in a very large surface area, as opposed to a chocolate bar that has a very small relative surface area. The small, surface area form dramatically increases solubility. Decreasing the solvent (most of the time, water) will decrease solubility.

13. A: The quantity of a solute in a solution can be calculated by multiplying the molarity of the solution by the volume. The equivalence point is the point at which an unknown solute has completely reacted with a known solute concentration. The limiting reactant is the reactant completely consumed by a reaction. The theoretical yield is the quantity of product produced by a reaction.

14. A: When salt is added to water, it increases its boiling point. This is an example of a colligative property, which is any property that changes the physical property of a substance. This particular colligative property of boiling point elevation occurs because the extra solute dissolved in water reduces the surface area of the water, impeding it from vaporizing. If heat is applied, though, it gives water particles enough kinetic energy to vaporize. This additional heat results in an increased boiling point.

Other colligative properties of solutions include the following: their melting points decrease with the addition of solute, and their osmotic pressure increases (because it creates a concentration gradient that was otherwise not there).

15. C: Pressure has little effect on the solubility of a liquid solution because liquid is not easily compressible; therefore, increased pressure won't result in increased kinetic energy. Pressure increases solubility in gaseous solutions, since it causes them to move faster.

16. B: Nonpolar molecules have hydrophobic regions that do not dissolve in water. Oil is a nonpolar molecule that repels water. Polar molecules combine readily with water, which is, itself, a polar solvent. Polar molecules are hydrophilic or "water-loving" because their polar regions have intermolecular bonding with water via hydrogen bonds. Some structures and molecules are both polar and nonpolar, like the phospholipid bilayer. The phospholipid bilayer has polar heads that are the external "water-loving portions" and hydrophobic tails that are immiscible in water. Polar solvents dissolve polar solutes, and nonpolar solvents dissolve nonpolar solutes. One way to remember these is "Like dissolves like."

17. A: A catalyst increases the rate of a chemical reaction by lowering the activation energy. Enzymes are biological protein catalysts that are utilized by organisms to facilitate anabolic and catabolic reactions. They speed up the rate of reaction by making the reaction easier (perhaps by orienting a molecule more favorably upon induced fit, for example). Catalysts are not used up by the reaction and can be used over and over again.

18. C: Proteins are made up of chains of amino acids. Lipids are usually nonpolar, hydrophobic molecules. Nucleic acids are made of nucleotides. Carbohydrates are ring-like molecules built using carbon, oxygen, and hydrogen.

19. C: 2: 9:10:4. These are the coefficients that follow the law of conservation of matter. The coefficient times the subscript of each element should be the same on both sides of the equation.

20. A: Ionic bonding is the result of electrons transferred between atoms. When an atom loses one or more electrons, a cation, or positively-charged ion, is formed. An anion, or negatively-charged ion, is formed when an atom gains one or more electrons. Ionic bonds are formed from the attraction between a positively-charged cation and a negatively-charged anion. The bond between sodium and chloride in table salt or sodium chloride, Na^+Cl^-, is an example of an ionic bond.

21. A: Oxidation is when a substance loses electrons in a chemical reaction, and reduction is when a substance gains electrons. Any element by itself has a charge of 0, as iron and oxygen do on the reactant side. In the ionic compound formed, iron has a +3 charge, and oxygen has a -2 charge. Because iron had a zero charge that then changed to +3, it means that it lost three electrons and was oxidized. Oxygen that gained two electrons was reduced.

22. C: Fission occurs when heavy nuclei are split and is currently the energy source that fuels power plants. Fusion, on the other hand, is the combining of small nuclei and produces far more energy, and it is the nuclear reaction that powers stars like the sun. Harnessing the extreme energy released by fusion has proven impossible so far, which is unfortunate since its waste products are not radioactive, while waste produced by fission typically is.

23. A: Alpha decay involves a helium particle emission (with two neutrons). Beta decay involves emission of an electron or positron, and gamma is just high-energy light emissions.

24. B: Choice *A* is false because it is possible to have a very strong acid with a pH between 0 and 1. *C* is false because the pH scale is from 0 to 14, and -2 is outside the boundaries. *D* is false because a solution with a pH of 2 has ten times fewer hydronium ions than a pH of 1 solution.

25. C: Gamma is the lightest radioactive decay with the most energy, and this high energy is toxic to cells. Due to its weightlessness, gamma rays are extremely penetrating. Alpha particles are heavy and can be easily shielded by skin. Beta particles are electrons and can penetrate more than an alpha particle because they are lighter. Beta particles can be shielded by plastic.

Anatomy and Physiology

General Terminology

Anatomy may be defined as the structural makeup of an organism. The study of anatomy may be divided into microscopic/fine anatomy and macroscopic/gross anatomy. **Fine anatomy** concerns itself with viewing the features of the body with the aid of a microscope, while **gross anatomy** concerns itself with viewing the features of the body with the naked eye. **Physiology** refers to the functions of an organism and it examines the chemical or physical functions that help the body function appropriately.

Levels of Organization of the Human Body

All the parts of the human body are built of individual units called **cells.** Groups of similar cells are arranged into **tissues**, different tissues are arranged into **organs,** and organs working together form entire **organ systems**. The human body has twelve organ systems that govern circulation, digestion, immunity, hormones, movement, support, coordination, urination & excretion, reproduction (male and female), respiration, and general protection.

Body Cavities

The body is partitioned into different hollow spaces that house organs. The human body contains the following cavities:

- **Cranial cavity:** The cranial cavity is surrounded by the skull and contains organs such as the brain and pituitary gland.

- **Thoracic cavity:** The thoracic cavity is encircled by the sternum (breastbone) and ribs. It contains organs such as the lungs, heart, trachea (windpipe), esophagus, and bronchial tubes.

- **Abdominal cavity:** The abdominal cavity is separated from the thoracic cavity by the diaphragm. It contains organs such as the stomach, gallbladder, liver, small intestines, and large intestines. The abdominal organs are held in place by a membrane called the peritoneum.

- **Pelvic cavity:** The pelvic cavity is enclosed by the pelvis, or bones of the hip. It contains organs such as the urinary bladder, urethra, ureters, anus, and rectum. It contains the reproductive organs as well. In females, the pelvic cavity also contains the uterus.

- **Spinal cavity:** The spinal cavity is surrounded by the vertebral column. The vertebral column has five regions: cervical, thoracic, lumbar, sacral, and coccygeal. The spinal cord runs through the middle of the spinal cavity.

Three Primary Body Planes

A **plane** is an imaginary flat surface. The three primary planes of the human body are frontal, sagittal, and transverse. The **frontal**, or **coronal,** plane is a vertical plane that divides the body or organ into front (anterior) and back (posterior) portions. The **sagittal,** or **lateral,** plane is a vertical plane divides the body or organ into right and left sides. The **transverse**, or **axial**, plane is a horizontal plane that divides the body or organ into upper and lower portions. In medical imaging, computed tomography (CT) scans are oriented only in the transverse plane; while magnetic resonance imaging (MRI) scans may be oriented in any of the three planes.

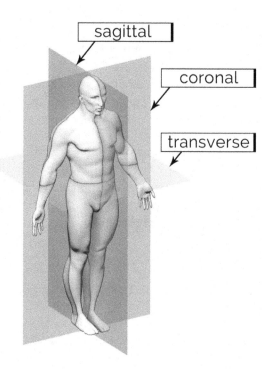

Note the body above is in the **anatomic position**. In anatomic position, the body and head are straight up and down, the feet are close but not touching, and the hands are pointed forward.

<u>Terms of Direction</u>
Medial refers to a structure being closer to the midline of the body. For example, the nose is medial to the eyes.

Lateral refers to a structure being farther from the midline of the body, and it is the opposite of medial. For example, the eyes are lateral to the nose.

Proximal refers to a structure or body part located near an attachment point. For example, the elbow is proximal to the wrist.

Distal refers to a structure or body part located far from an attachment point, and it is the opposite of proximal. For example, the wrist is distal to the elbow.

Anterior means toward the front in humans. For example, the lips are anterior to the teeth. The term **ventral** can be used in place of anterior.

Posterior means toward the back in humans, and it is the opposite of anterior. For example, the teeth are posterior to the lips. The term **dorsal** can be used in place of posterior.

Superior means above and refers to a structure closer to the head. For example, the head is superior to the neck. The terms **cephalic** or **cranial** may be used in place of superior.

Inferior means below and refers to a structure farther from the head, and it is the opposite of superior. For example, the neck is inferior to the head. The term **caudal** may be used in place of inferior.

Superficial refers to a structure closer to the surface. For example, the muscles are superficial because they are just beneath the surface of the skin.

Deep refers to a structure farther from the surface, and it is the opposite of superficial. For example, the femur is a deep structure lying beneath the muscles.

Body Regions
Terms for general locations on the body include:
- Cervical: relating to the neck
- Clavicular: relating to the clavicle, or collarbone
- Ocular: relating to the eyes
- Acromial: relating to the shoulder
- Cubital: relating to the elbow
- Brachial: relating to the arm
- Carpal: relating to the wrist
- Thoracic: relating to the chest
- Abdominal: relating to the abdomen
- Pubic: relating to the groin
- Pelvic: relating to the pelvis, or bones of the hip
- Femoral: relating to the femur, or thigh bone
- Geniculate: relating to the knee
- Pedal: relating to the foot
- Palmar: relating to the palm of the hand
- Plantar: relating to the sole of the foot

Abdominopelvic Regions and Quadrants
The **abdominopelvic region** may be defined as the combination of the abdominal and the pelvic cavities. The region's upper border is the breasts and its lower border is the groin region. The region is divided into the following nine sections:

- Right hypochondriac: region below the cartilage of the ribs
- Epigastric: region above the stomach between the hypochondriac regions
- Left hypochondriac: region below the cartilage of the ribs
- Right lumbar: region of the waist
- Umbilical: region between the lumbar regions where the umbilicus, or belly button (navel), is located
- Left lumbar: region of the waist
- Right inguinal: region of the groin
- Hypogastric: region below the stomach between the inguinal regions
- Left inguinal: region of the groin

A simpler way to describe the abdominopelvic area would be to divide it into the following quadrants:

- Right upper quadrant (RUQ): Encompasses the right hypochondriac, right lumbar, epigastric, and umbilical regions.

- Right lower quadrant (RLQ): Encompasses the right lumbar, right inguinal, hypogastric, and umbilical regions.

- Left upper quadrant (LUQ): Encompasses the left hypochondriac, left lumbar, epigastric, and umbilical regions.

- Left lower quadrant (LLQ): Encompasses the left lumbar, left inguinal, hypogastric, and umbilical regions.

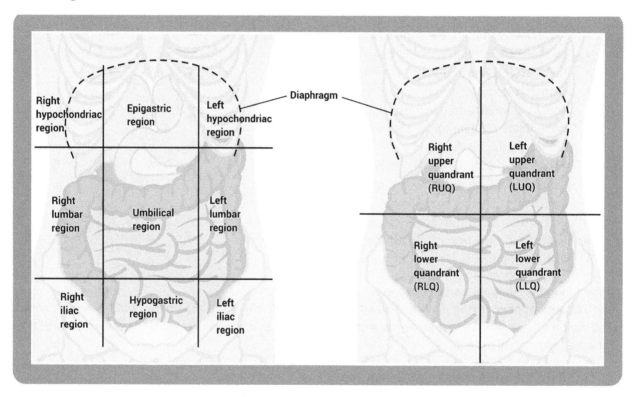

Histology

Histology is the examination of specialized cells and cell groups that perform a specific function by working together. Although there are trillions of cells in the human body, there are only 200 different types of cells. Groups of cells form biological tissues, and tissues combine to form organs, such as the heart and kidney. Organs are structures that have many different functions that are vital to living creatures. There are four primary types of tissue: epithelial, connective, muscle, and neural. Each tissue type has specific characteristics that enable organs and organ systems to function properly.

Muscle: Muscle tissue supports the body and allows it to move, and muscles are special as their cells have the ability to contract. There are three distinct types of muscle tissue: skeletal, smooth, and cardiac. **Skeletal muscle** is voluntary, or under conscious control, and is usually attached to bones. Most body movement is directly caused by the contraction of skeletal muscle. **Smooth muscle** is typically involuntary, or not under conscious control, and may be found in blood vessels, the walls of hollow organs, and the urinary bladder. **Cardiac muscle** is involuntary and found in the heart, which helps propel blood throughout the body.

Nervous: Nervous tissue is unique in that it is able to coordinate information from sensory organs as well as communicate the proper behavioral responses. **Neurons,** or nerve cells, are the workhorses of the nervous system. They communicate via **action potentials** (electrical signals) and **neurotransmitters** (chemical signals).

Epithelial: Epithelial tissue covers the external surfaces of organs and lines many of the body's cavities. Epithelial tissue helps to protect the body from invasion by microbes (bacteria, viruses, parasites), fluid loss, and injury.

Epithelial cell shapes can be:

- Squamous: cells with a flat shape
- Cuboidal: cells with a cubed shape
- Columnar: cells shaped like a column

Epithelial cells can be arranged in four patterns:

- Simple: a type of epithelium composed solely from a single layer of cells
- Stratified: a type of epithelium composed of multiple layers of cells
- Pseudostratified: a type of epithelium which appears to be stratified but in reality consists of only one layer of cells
- Transitional: a type of epithelium noted for its ability to expand and contract

Connective: Connective tissue supports and connects the tissues and organs of the body. Connective tissue is composed of cells dispersed throughout a matrix which can be gel, liquid, protein fibers, or salts. The primary protein fibers in the matrix are collagen (for strength), elastin (for flexibility), and reticulum (for support). Connective tissue can be categorized as either **loose** or **dense.** Examples of connective tissue include bones, cartilage, ligaments, tendons, blood, and adipose (fat) tissue.

Mitosis and Meiosis

The **cell cycle** is the process by which a cell divides and duplicates itself. There are two processes by which a cell can divide itself: mitosis and meiosis. In **mitosis,** the daughter cells that are produced from parental cell division are identical to each other and the parent. **Meiosis** is a unique process that involves two stages of cell division and produces haploid cells, which are cells containing only one set of chromosomes, from diploid parent cells, which are cells containing two sets of chromosomes.

Skin

The **integumentary system** includes skin, hair, nails, oil glands, and sweat glands. The largest organ of the integumentary system (and of the body), the skin, acts as a barrier and protects the body from mechanical impact, variations in temperature, microorganisms, chemicals, and UV radiation from the sun. It regulates body temperature, peripheral circulation, and excretes waste through sweat. It also contains a large network of nerve cells that relay changes in the external environment to the brain.

<u>Layers of Skin</u>
Skin consists of two layers, the surface **epidermis** and the inner **dermis**. The subcutaneous **hypodermis** is below the dermis and contains a layer of fat and connective tissue that are both important for insulation.

The whole epidermis is composed of epithelial cells that lack blood vessels. The outer epidermis is composed of dead cells which surround the living cells underneath. The most inner epidermal tissue is a single layer of cells called the **stratum basale** which is composed of rapidly dividing cells that push old cells to the skin's surface. When being pushed out, the cells' organelles disappear, and they start producing a protein called **keratin** that eventually forms a tough waterproof layer. This outer layer sloughs off every four to five weeks. The **melanocytes** in the stratum basale produce the pigment melanin that absorbs UV rays and protects the skin. Skin also produces vitamin D if exposed to sunlight.

The dermis underneath the epidermis contains supporting collagen fibers peppered with nerves, blood vessels, hair follicles, sweat glands, oil glands, and smooth muscles.

<u>Skin's Involvement in Temperature Homeostasis</u>
The skin has a thermoregulatory role in the human body that is controlled by a negative feedback loop. The control center of temperature regulation is the hypothalamus in the brain. When the hypothalamus is alerted by receptors from the dermis, it secretes hormones that activate effectors to keep internal temperature at a set point of 98.6°F (37°C). If the environment is too cold, the hypothalamus will initiate a pathway that induces muscle shivering to release heat energy as well as constrict blood vessels to limit heat loss. In hot conditions, the hypothalamus will initiate a pathway that vasodilates blood vessels to increase heat loss and stimulate sweating for evaporative cooling. Evaporative cooling occurs when the hottest water particles evaporate and leave behind the coolest ones. This cools down the body.

<u>Sebaceous Glands vs. Sweat Glands</u>
The skin also contains oil glands, or **sebaceous glands**, and sweat glands that are **exocrine** because their substances are secreted through ducts. **Endocrine** glands secrete substances into the blood stream instead. Oil glands are attached to hair follicles. They secrete **sebum**, an oily substance that moisturizes the skin, protecting it from water loss. Sebum also keeps the skin elastic. Also, sebum's slight acidity provides a chemical defense against bacterial and fungal infections.

Sweat glands not attached to hair follicles are called **eccrine** glands. They are all over the body and these are the ones responsible for thermoregulation. They also remove bodily waste by secreting water and electrolytes. Sweat glands attached to hair follicles are apocrine glands and there are not nearly as many. **Apocrine** glands are only active post-puberty. They secrete a thicker, viscous substance that is attractive to bacteria, leading to the unpleasant smell in armpits, feet, and the groin. They are stimulated during stress and arousal.

Skeletal System

<u>Axial Skeleton and Appendicular Skeleton</u>
The skeletal system is composed of 206 bones interconnected by tough connective tissue called ligaments. The **axial skeleton** can be considered the north-south axis of the skeleton. It includes the spinal column, sternum, ribs, and skull. There are 80 bones in the axial skeleton, and 33 of them are vertebrae. The ribs make up 12 of the bones in the axial skeleton.

The remaining 126 bones are in the **appendicular skeleton**, which contains bones of the appendages like the collarbone (clavicle), shoulders (scapula), arms, hands, hips, legs, and feet. The arm bones consist of the upper humerus with the radius and ulna that attach to the hands. The wrists, hands, and fingers are composed of the carpals, metacarpals, and phalanges, respectively. The femur attaches to the hips. The patella or kneecap connects the femur to the fibula and tibia. The ankles, feet, and toes are composed of the tarsals, metatarsals, and phalanges, respectively.

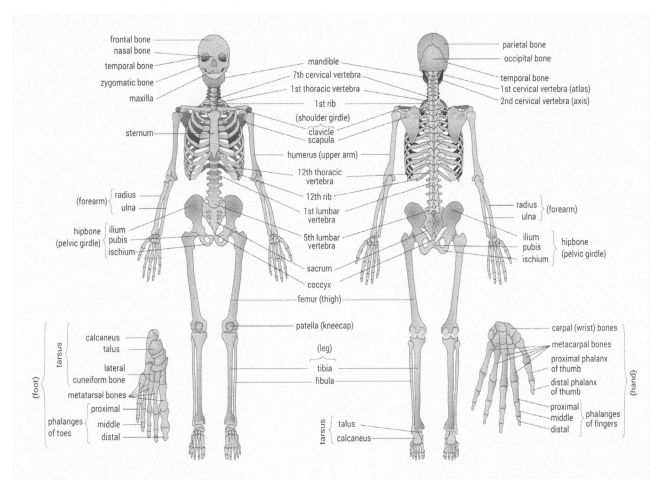

Functions of the Skeletal System

One of the skeletal system's most important functions is to protect vital internal organs. The skull protects the brain, the ribs protect the lungs and heart, the vertebrae protect the spinal column, and the pelvis protects the uterus and other reproductive organs. Yellow bone marrow stores lipids, or fats. Red bone marrow produces red and white blood cells as well as platelets in a process known as **hemopoiesis**. The bones themselves store the essential minerals calcium and phosphorous. The organization of the skeleton allows us to stand upright and acts as a foundation for organs and tissues to attach and maintain their location. This is similar to how the wooden frame of a house has room partitions to designate the type of room and floors that furniture can attach to.

The skeletal system and the muscular system are literally interconnected and allow for voluntary movement. Strong connective tissues called **tendons** attach bones to muscles. Most muscles work in opposing pairs and act as levers. For example, flexing the biceps brings the arm bones together and flexing the triceps pushes them apart. **Synovial joints** are movable joints, and they are rich with cartilage, connective tissue, and synovial fluid which acts as a lubricant. The majority of joints are synovial joints, and they include hinge joints, like the one at the elbow, which allows for opening and closing.

The vertebrae are **cartilaginous joints** which have spaces between them filled with cushion-like discs that act as shock absorbers and glue that holds the vertebrae together. The reason for the tight packing of the vertebrae is to protect the spinal cord inside. This limits their movement, but because there are so many of them it allows the backbone to be flexible.

Fibrous joints like those in the skull have fibrous tissue between the bones and no cavity between them. These are fixed joints that are immobile.

Compact and Spongy Bone

Osteoclasts, osteoblasts, and osteocytes are the three types of bone cells. **Osteoclasts** break down old bone, **osteoblasts** make new bone, and **osteocytes** are the mature functional bone cells. Bone is constantly regenerating due to the osteoblasts/osteoclasts that line all types of bones and the blood vessels inside them. The cells all exist within a matrix of collagen fibers that provide resistance to tension and minerals that provide resistance to compression. Because of the collagen and mineral matrix, bones have ample reinforcement to collectively support the entire human body.

Bones can be classified as any of the following:

- **Long bones** include tube-like rods like the arm and leg bones.
- **Short bones** are tube-like rods that are smaller than long bones like the fingers and toes.
- **Flat bones** are thin and flat like the ribs and breastbone.
- **Irregular bones** like the vertebrae are compact and don't fit into the other categories.

The outer tissue of the bone is surrounded by connective tissue known as **periosteum**. It appears shiny, smooth, and white. It protects the bone, anchors the bone to the connective tissue that surrounds muscles, and links the bone to the circulatory and nervous system. **Compact bone** is underneath the periosteum and is made of a dense blend of tightly packed osteocytes a mineral reservoir of calcium and phosphorous. Compact bones have a **Haversian system** that is composed of embedded blood vessels, lymph vessels, and nerve bundles that span the interior of the bone from one end to the other. Branching from the central canal to the surface of the bone are the **canals of Volkmann,** which deliver materials to peripheral osteocytes. Concentric circles surround the central Haversian canal, and these **lamallae** have gaps between them called **lacunae** where osteocytes are embedded.

In contrast, **spongy bone** is very porous and more flexible than compact bone. It is at the ends of long bones and the central part of flat bones. It looks like a honeycomb, and the open spaces are connected by **trabeculae** which are beams of tissue that add support. They add strength without adding mass.

Cartilage is a very flexible connective tissue made of collagen and the flexible elastin. It has no blood vessels and obtains materials via diffusion. It is replaced by bone starting in infancy in a process called **ossification**.

Muscular System

The muscular system is responsible for involuntary and voluntary movement of the body. There are three types of muscle: skeletal, cardiac, and smooth.

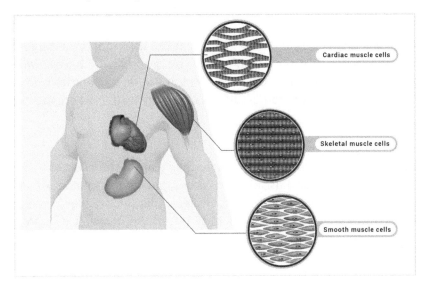

Skeletal Muscles

Skeletal muscles, or **voluntary muscles**, are attached to bones by tendons and are responsible for voluntary movement. The connecting tendons are made up of dense bands of connective tissue and have collagen fibers that firmly attach the muscle to the bone. Their fibers are actually woven into the coverings of the bone and muscle so that they can withstand pressure and tension. They usually work in opposing pairs like the bicep and tricep, for example. Muscles that work together are called **synergists.**

Skeletal muscles are made of bundles of long **fibers** that are composed of cells with many nuclei due to their length. These fibers contain **myofibrils,** and myofibrils are made of alternating **filaments**. The thicker myosin filaments are in between the smaller actin filaments in a unit called a **sarcomere**, and the overlapping regions give the muscle their characteristic striated, or striped, appearance. Actin filaments are attached to exterior Z lines, myosin filaments are attached to a central M line, and when a muscle is at rest, there is a gap between the Z line and the myosin filaments. Only when the muscle contracts and the actin filaments slide over the myosin filaments does the myosin reach the Z line, as illustrated in the picture below. This **sliding-filament model of muscle contraction** is dependent on myosin molecules forming and breaking cross-bridges with actin in order to pull the actin filaments closer to the M line.

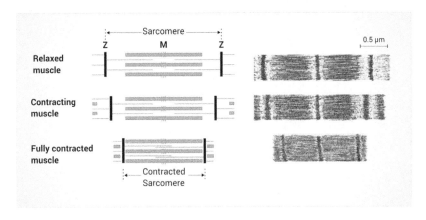

Skeletal muscles are controlled by the nervous system. Motor neurons connect to muscle fibers via neuromuscular junctions. Motor neurons must release the neurotransmitter **acetylcholine**, which releases calcium ions to stimulate myosin cross-bridging and contraction. As the acetylcholine stops being released, the contraction ends.

Smooth Muscles
Smooth muscles are responsible for involuntary movement like food moving through the digestive tract and blood moving through vessels. They have only one nucleus and do not have striations because actin and myosin filaments do not have an organized arrangement like skeletal muscles do. Unlike skeletal muscle, these muscles don't require neuromuscular junctions. Instead, they operate via gap junctions which send impulses directly from cell to cell.

Cardiac Muscles
Cardiac muscle cells are found only in the heart where they control the heart's rhythm and blood pressure. Like skeletal muscle, cardiac muscle has striations, but cardiac muscle cells are smaller than skeletal muscle cells, so they typically have only one nucleus. Like smooth muscle, cardiac muscles do not require neurotransmitter release by motor neurons to function, and they instead operate via gap junctions.

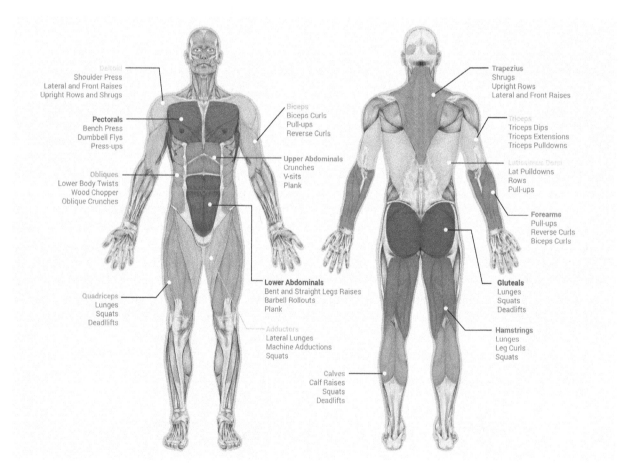

Nervous System

The human nervous system coordinates the body's response to stimuli from inside and outside the body. There are two major types of nervous system cells: neurons and neuroglia. **Neurons** are the workhorses of the nervous system and form a complex communication network that transmits electrical impulses termed **action potentials**, while **neuroglia** connect and support them. Motor neurons use sodium and potassium pumps and channels in order to make action potentials occur.

Although some neurons monitor the senses, some control muscles, and some connect the brain to others, all neurons have four common characteristics:

- **Dendrites:** These receive electrical signals from other neurons across small gaps called *synapses*.
- **Nerve cell body:** This is the hub of processing and protein manufacture for the neuron.
- **Axon:** This transmits the signal from the cell body to other neurons.
- **Terminals:** These bridge the neuron to dendrites of other neurons and deliver the signal via chemical messengers called **neurotransmitters.**

Here an illustration of this:

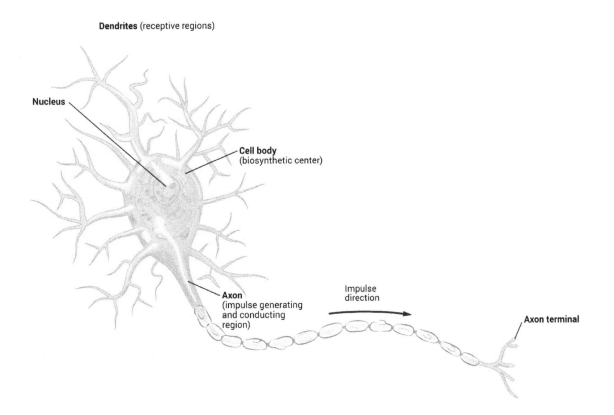

There are two major divisions of the nervous system: central and peripheral:

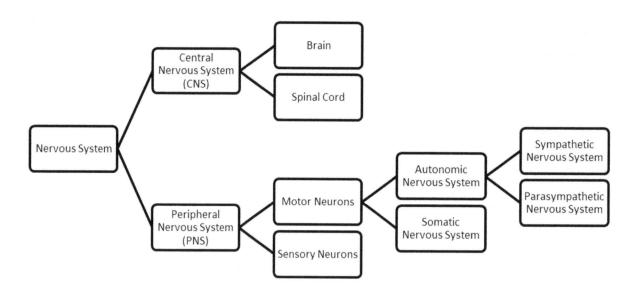

Central Nervous System

The **central nervous system (CNS)** consists of the brain and spinal cord. Three layers of membranes called the meninges cover and separate the CNS from the rest of the body.

The major divisions of the brain are the forebrain, the midbrain, and the hindbrain.

The **forebrain** consists of the cerebrum, the thalamus and hypothalamus, and the rest of the limbic system. The **cerebrum** is the largest part of the brain, and its most well-documented part is the outer cerebral cortex. The cerebrum is divided into right and left hemispheres, and each cerebral cortex hemisphere has four discrete areas, or lobes: frontal, temporal, parietal, and occipital.

The **frontal lobe** governs duties such as voluntary movement, judgment, problem solving, and planning, while the other lobes are more sensory. The **temporal lobe** integrates hearing and language comprehension, the **parietal lobe** processes sensory input from the skin, and the **occipital lobe** functions to process visual input from the eyes. For completeness, the other two senses, smell and taste, are processed via the olfactory bulbs. The thalamus helps organize and coordinate all of this sensory input in a meaningful way for the brain to interpret.

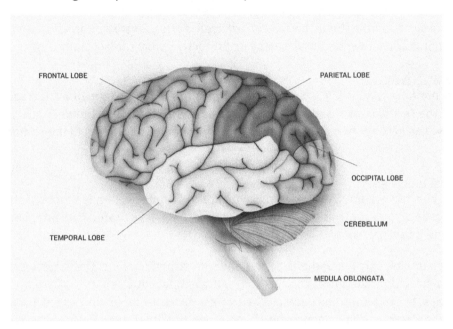

The **hypothalamus** controls the endocrine system and all of the hormones that govern long-term effects on the body. Each hemisphere of the limbic system includes a **hippocampus** (which plays a vital role in memory), an **amygdala** (which is involved with emotional responses like fear and anger), and other small bodies and nuclei associated with memory and pleasure.

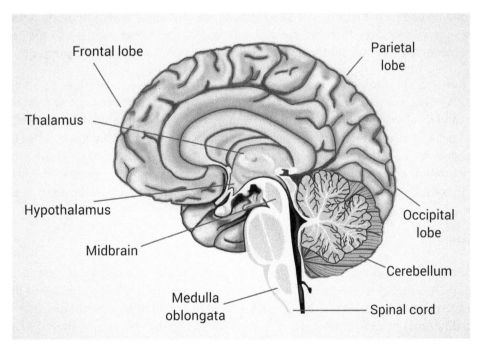

The **midbrain** is in charge of alertness, sleep/wake cycles, and temperature regulation, and it includes the **substantia nigra** which produces melatonin to regulate sleep patterns. The notable components of the **hindbrain** include the **medulla oblongata** and **cerebellum.** The medulla oblongata is located just above the spinal cord and is responsible for crucial involuntary functions such as breathing, heart rate, swallowing, and the regulation of blood pressure. Together with other parts of the hindbrain, the midbrain and medulla oblongata form the **brain stem.** The brain stem connects the spinal cord to the rest of the brain. To the rear of the brain stem sits the cerebellum, which plays key roles in posture, balance, and muscular coordination. The spinal cord itself carries sensory information to the brain and motor information to the body, encapsulated by its protective bony spinal column.

Peripheral Nervous System

The **peripheral nervous system (PNS)** includes all nervous tissue besides the brain and spinal cord. The PNS consists of the sets of cranial and spinal nerves and relays information between the CNS and the rest of the body. The PNS has two divisions: the autonomic nervous system and the somatic nervous system.

Autonomic Nervous System

The **autonomic nervous system (ANS)** governs involuntary, or reflexive, body functions. Ultimately, the autonomic nervous system controls functions such as breathing, heart rate, digestion, body temperature, and blood pressure.

The ANS is split between parasympathetic nerves and sympathetic nerves. These two nerve types are antagonistic and have opposite effects on the body. **Parasympathetic** nerves typically are useful when resting or during safe conditions and decrease heart rate, decrease inhalation speed, prepare digestion, and allow urination and excretion. **Sympathetic** nerves, on the other hand, become active when a person is under stress or excited, and they increase heart rate, increase breathing rates, and inhibit digestion, urination, and excretion.

Somatic Nervous System and the Reflex Arc

The **somatic nervous system (SNS)** governs the conscious, or voluntary, control of skeletal muscles and their corresponding body movements. The SNS contains afferent and efferent neurons. **Afferent** neurons carry sensory messages from the skeletal muscles, skin, or sensory organs to the CNS. **Efferent neurons relay motor messages from the CNS to skeletal muscles, skin, or sensory organs.**

The SNS also has a role in involuntary movements called **reflexes**. A reflex is defined as an involuntary response to a stimulus. They are transmitted via what is termed a **reflex arc**, where a stimulus is sensed by an affector and its afferent neuron, interpreted and rerouted by an interneuron, and delivered to effector muscles by an efferent neuron where they respond to the initial stimulus. A reflex is able to bypass the brain by being rerouted through the spinal cord; the interneuron decides the proper course of action rather than the brain. The reflex arc results in an instantaneous, involuntary response. For example, a physician tapping on the knee produces an involuntary knee jerk referred to as the patellar tendon reflex.

Endocrine System

The **endocrine system** is made up of the ductless tissues and glands that secrete hormones directly into the bloodstream. It is similar to the nervous system in that it controls various functions of the body, but it does so via secretion of hormones in the bloodstream as opposed to nerve impulses. The endocrine system is also different because its effects last longer than that of the nervous system. Nerve impulses are immediate while hormone responses can last for minutes or even days.

The endocrine system works closely with the nervous system to regulate the physiological activities of the other systems of the body in order to maintain homeostasis. Hormone secretions are controlled by tight feedback loops that are generally regulated by the hypothalamus, the bridge between the nervous and endocrine systems. The hypothalamus receives sensory input via the nervous system and responds by stimulating or inhibiting the pituitary gland which stimulates or inhibits several other glands. The tight control is due to hormone secretions.

Hormones are chemicals that bind to specific target cells. Each hormone will only bind to a target cell that has a specific receptor that has the correct shape. For example, testosterone will not attach to skin cells because skin cells have no receptor that recognizes testosterone.

There are two types of hormones: steroid and protein. Steroid hormones are lipid, nonpolar substances, and most are able to diffuse across cell membranes. Once they do, they bind to a receptor that initiates a signal transduction cascade that affects gene expression. Non-steroid hormones bind to receptors on cell membranes that also initiate a signal transduction cascade that affects enzyme activity and chemical reactions.

Major Endocrine Glands

Hypothalamus: This gland is a part of the brain. It connects the nervous system to the endocrine system because it receives sensory information through nerves and it sends instructions via hormones delivered to the pituitary.

Pituitary Gland: This gland is pea-sized and is found at the bottom of the hypothalamus. It has two lobes called the anterior and posterior lobes. It plays an important role in regulating other endocrine glands. For example, it secretes growth hormone which regulates growth. Other hormones that are released by this gland control the reproductive system, childbirth, nursing, blood osmolarity, and metabolism.

The hormones and glands respond to each other via feedback loops, and a typical feedback loop is illustrated in the picture below. The hypothalamus and pituitary gland are master controllers of most of the other glands.

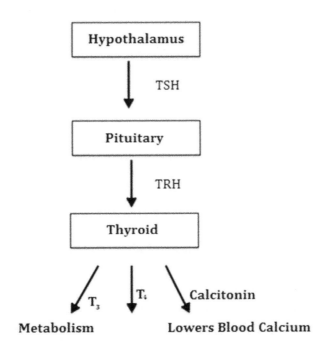

Thymus Gland: This gland is located in the chest cavity, embedded in connective tissue. It produces several hormones that are important for development and maintenance of T lymphocytes, which are important cells for immunity.

Adrenal Gland: One adrenal gland is attached to the top of each kidney. It produces epinephrine and norepinephrine which cause the "fight or flight" response in the face of danger or stress. These hormones raise heart rate, blood pressure, dilate bronchioles, and deliver blood to the muscles. All of these actions increase circulation and release glucose so that the body has an energy burst.

Pineal Gland: The pineal gland secretes melatonin, which is a hormone that regulates the body's circadian rhythms which are the natural wake-sleep cycles.

Testes and Ovaries: They secrete testosterone and both estrogen and progesterone, respectively. They are responsible for secondary sex characteristics, gamete development, and female hormones are important for embryonic development.

Thyroid Gland: This gland releases hormones like thyroxine and calcitonin. Thyroxine stimulates metabolism, and calcitonin monitors the amount of circulating calcium. Calcitonin signals the body to regulating calcium from bone reserves as well as kidney reabsorption of calcium.

Parathyroid Glands: These are four pea-sized glands located on the posterior surface of the thyroid. The main hormone that is secreted is called parathyroid hormone (PTH) which influences calcium levels like calcitonin, except it is antagonistic. PTH increases extracellular levels of calcium while calcitonin decreases it.

Pancreas: The pancreas is an organ that has both endocrine and exocrine functions. It functions outside of a typical feedback loop in that blood sugar seems to signal the pancreas itself. The endocrine functions are controlled by the pancreatic **islets of Langerhans**, which are groups of beta cells scattered throughout the gland that secrete insulin to lower blood sugar levels in the body. Neighboring alpha cells secrete glucagon to raise blood sugar. These complementary hormones keep blood sugar in check.

Circulatory System

The **cardiovascular system** (also called the **circulatory system**) is a network of organs and tubes that transport blood, hormones, nutrients, oxygen, and other gases to cells and tissues throughout the body. It is also known as the cardiovascular system. The major components of the circulatory system are the blood vessels, blood, and heart.

Blood Vessels
In the circulatory system, **blood vessels** are responsible for transporting blood throughout the body. The three major types of blood vessels in the circulatory system are arteries, veins, and capillaries. **Arteries** carry blood from the heart to the rest of the body. **Veins** carry blood from the body to the heart. **Capillaries** connect arteries to veins and form networks that exchange materials between the blood and the cells.

In general, arteries are stronger and thicker than veins, as they withstand high pressures exerted by the blood as the heart pumps it through the body. Arteries control blood flow through either **vasoconstriction** (narrowing of the blood vessel's diameter) or **vasodilation** (widening of the blood vessel's diameter). The smallest arteries, which are farthest from the heart, are called **arterioles.** The blood in veins is under much lower pressures, so veins have valves to prevent the backflow of blood.

Most of the exchange between the blood and tissues takes place through the capillaries. There are three types of capillaries: continuous, fenestrated, and sinusoidal.

Continuous capillaries are made up of epithelial cells tightly connected together. As a result, they limit the types of materials that pass into and out of the blood. Continuous capillaries are the most common type of capillary. **Fenestrated capillaries** have openings that allow materials to be freely exchanged between the blood and tissues. They are commonly found in the digestive, endocrine, and urinary systems. **Sinusoidal capillaries** have larger openings and allow proteins and blood cells through. They are found primarily in the liver, bone marrow, and spleen.

Blood

Blood is vital to the human body. It is a liquid connective tissue that serves as a transport system for supplying cells with nutrients and carrying away their wastes. The average adult human has five to six quarts of blood circulating through their body. Approximately 55% of blood is plasma (the fluid portion), and the remaining 45% is composed of solid cells and cell parts. There are three major types of blood cells:

- Red blood cells, or **erythrocytes**, transport oxygen throughout the body. They contain a protein called **hemoglobin** that allows them to carry oxygen. The iron in the hemoglobin gives the cells and the blood their red colors.

- White blood cells, or **leukocytes**, are responsible for fighting infectious diseases and maintaining the immune system. Monocytes, lymphocytes (including B-cells and T-cells), neutrophils, basophils, and eosinophils compose the white blood cells. All are developed in bone marrow. **Monocytes** eat and destroy invaders like bacteria and viruses. **Lymphocytes** are responsible for antibody creation in the defense against invasive organisms and infections. **Neutrophils**, the most abundant white blood cell, take out bacterial and fungal organisms. They are the first line of defense against infections. **Basophils** and mast cells secrete histamine, the substance responsible for itching associated with allergic diseases. **Eosinophils** target parasites and cancer cells, and are part of the body's allergic response. They have low phagocytic activity and primarily secrete destructive enzymes.

- **Platelets** are cell fragments which play a central role in the blood clotting process.

All blood cells in adults are produced in the bone marrow—red blood cells from red marrow and white blood cells from yellow marrow.

Heart

The **heart** is a two-part, muscular pump that forcefully pushes blood throughout the human body. The human heart has four chambers—two upper atria and two lower ventricles, a pair on the left and a pair on the right. Anatomically, *left* and *right* correspond to the sides of the body that the patient themselves would refer to as left and right.

Four valves help to section off the chambers from one another. Between the right atrium and ventricle, the three flaps of the **tricuspid valve** keep blood from backflowing from the ventricle to the atrium, similar to how the two flaps of the **mitral valve** work between the left atrium and ventricle. As these two valves lie between an atrium and a ventricle, they are referred to as **atrioventricular (AV) valves**. The other two valves are **semilunar (SL)** and control blood flow into the two great arteries leaving the ventricles. The **pulmonary valve** connects the right ventricle to the pulmonary artery while the **aortic valve** connects the left ventricle to the aorta.

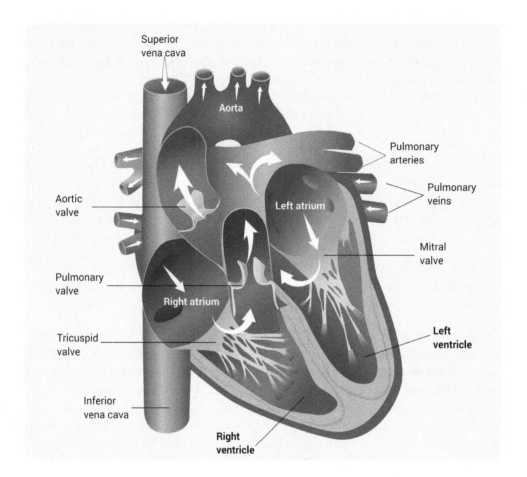

Cardiac Cycle

A **cardiac cycle** is one complete sequence of cardiac activity. The cardiac cycle represents the relaxation and contraction of the heart and can be divided into two phases: diastole and systole.

Diastole is the phase during which the heart relaxes and fills with blood. It gives rise to the diastolic blood pressure (DBP), which is the bottom number of a blood pressure reading. **Systole** is the phase during which the heart contracts and discharges blood. It gives rise to the systolic blood pressure (SBP), which is the top number of a blood pressure reading. The heart's electrical conduction system coordinates the cardiac cycle.

Types of Circulation

Five major blood vessels manage blood flow to and from the heart: the superior and inferior venae cavae, the aorta, the pulmonary artery, and the pulmonary vein.

The **superior vena cava** is a large vein that drains blood from the head and upper body. The **inferior vena cava** is a large vein that drains blood from the lower body. The **aorta** is the largest artery in the human body and carries blood from the heart to body tissues. The **pulmonary arteries** carry blood from the heart to the lungs. The **pulmonary veins** transport blood from the lungs to the heart.

In the human body, there are two types of circulation: pulmonary circulation and systemic circulation. **Pulmonary circulation** supplies blood to the lungs. Deoxygenated blood enters the right atrium of the heart and is routed through the tricuspid valve into the right ventricle. Deoxygenated blood then travels from the right ventricle of the heart through the pulmonary valve and into the pulmonary arteries. The pulmonary arteries carry the deoxygenated blood to the lungs. In the lungs, oxygen is absorbed, and carbon dioxide is released. The pulmonary veins carry oxygenated blood to the left atrium of the heart.

Systemic circulation supplies blood to all other parts of the body, except the lungs. Oxygenated blood flows from the left atrium of the heart through the mitral, or bicuspid, valve into the left ventricle of the heart. Oxygenated blood is then routed from the left ventricle of the heart through the aortic valve and into the aorta. The aorta delivers blood to the systemic arteries, which supply the body tissues. In the tissues, oxygen and nutrients are exchanged for carbon dioxide and other wastes. The deoxygenated blood along with carbon dioxide and wastes enter the systemic veins, where they are returned to the right atrium of the heart via the superior and inferior vena cava.

Respiratory System

The **respiratory system** enables breathing and supports the energy-making process in our cells. The respiratory system transports an essential reactant, oxygen, to cells so that they can produce energy in their mitochondria via cellular respiration. The respiratory system also removes carbon dioxide, a waste product of cellular respiration.

This system is divided into the upper respiratory system and the lower respiratory system. The **upper system** comprises the nose, the nasal cavity and sinuses, and the pharynx. The **lower respiratory system** comprises the larynx (voice box), the trachea (windpipe), the small passageways leading to the lungs, and the lungs.

The pathway of oxygen to the bloodstream begins with the nose and the mouth. Upon inhalation, air enters the nose and mouth and passes into the sinuses where it gets warmed, filtered, and humidified. The throat, or the pharynx, allows the entry of both food and air; however, only air moves into the trachea, or windpipe, since the epiglottis covers the trachea during swallowing and prevents food from entering. The trachea contains mucus and cilia. The mucus traps many airborne pathogens while the cilia act as bristles that sweep the pathogens away toward the top of the trachea where they are either swallowed or coughed out.

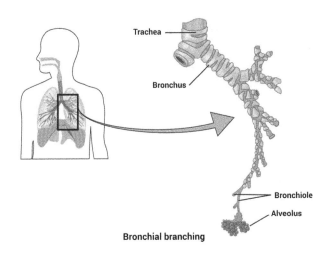

Trachea

Bronchus

Bronchiole

Alveolus

Bronchial branching

The **trachea** itself has two vocal cords at the top that make up the **larynx**. At its bottom, the trachea forks into two major **bronchi**—one for each lung. These bronchi continue to branch into smaller and smaller **bronchioles** before terminating in grape-like air sacs called **alveoli;** these alveoli are surrounded by capillaries and provide the body with an enormous amount of surface area to exchange oxygen and carbon dioxide gases, in a process called **external respiration**.

In total, the lungs contain about 1500 miles of airway passages. The right lung is divided into three lobes (superior, middle, and inferior), and the left lung is divided into two lobes (superior and inferior).

The left lung is smaller than the right lung, likely because it shares its space in the chest cavity with the heart.

A flat muscle underneath the lungs called the **diaphragm** controls breathing. When the diaphragm contracts, the volume of the chest cavity increases and indirectly decreases its air pressure. This decrease in air pressure creates a vacuum, and the lungs pull in air to fill the space. This difference in air pressure that pulls the air from outside of the body into the lungs in a process called negative pressure breathing.

Upon **inhalation** or **inspiration,** oxygen in the alveoli diffuses into the capillaries to be carried by blood to cells throughout the body, in a process called **internal respiration**. A protein called hemoglobin in red blood cells easily bonds with oxygen, removing it from the blood and allowing more oxygen to diffuse in. This protein allows the blood to take in 60 times more oxygen than the body could without it, and this explains how oxygen can become so concentrated in blood even though it is only 21% of the atmosphere. While oxygen diffuses from the alveoli into the capillaries, carbon dioxide diffuses from the capillaries into the alveoli. When the diaphragm relaxes, the elastic lungs snap back to their original shape; this decreases the volume of the chest cavity and increases the air pressure until it is back to normal. This increased air pressure pushes the carbon dioxide waste from the alveoli through **exhalation** or **expiration.**

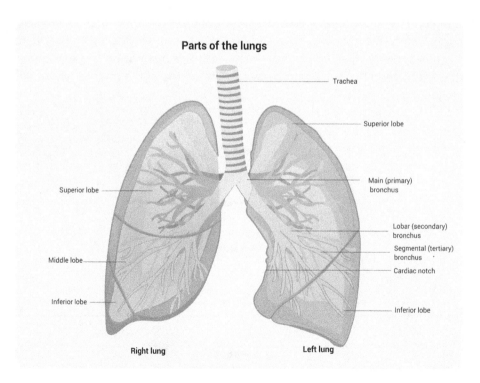

Parts of the lungs

Trachea

Superior lobe

Main (primary) bronchus

Lobar (secondary) bronchus

Segmental (tertiary) bronchus

Cardiac notch

Inferior lobe

Superior lobe

Middle lobe

Inferior lobe

Right lung

Left lung

The autonomic nervous system controls breathing. The medulla oblongata gets feedback regarding the carbon dioxide levels in the blood and will send a message to the diaphragm that it is time for a contraction. While breathing can be voluntary, it is mostly under autonomic control.

<u>Functions of the Respiratory System</u>
The respiratory system has many functions. Most importantly, it provides a large area for gas exchange between the air and the circulating blood. It protects the delicate respiratory surfaces from environmental variations and defends them against pathogens. It is responsible for producing the sounds that the body makes for speaking and singing, as well as for non-verbal communication. It also helps regulate blood volume and blood pressure by releasing vasopressin, and it is a regulator of blood pH due to its control over carbon dioxide release, as the aqueous form of carbon dioxide is the chief buffering agent in blood. Erythrocytes use carbonic anhydrase to convert most carbon dioxide in the blood to bicarbonate ions.

Digestive System

The human body relies completely on the **digestive system** to meet its nutritional needs. After food and drink are ingested, the digestive system breaks them down into their component nutrients and absorbs them so that the circulatory system can transport them to other cells to use for growth, energy, and cell repair. These nutrients may be classified as proteins, lipids, carbohydrates, vitamins, and minerals.

The digestive system is thought of chiefly in two parts: the **digestive tract** (also called the **alimentary tract** or **gastrointestinal tract**) and the accessory digestive organs. The digestive tract is the pathway in which food is ingested, digested, absorbed, and excreted. It is composed of the mouth, pharynx, esophagus, stomach, small and large intestines, rectum, and anus. **Peristalsis**, or wave-like contractions of smooth muscle, moves food and wastes through the digestive tract. The accessory digestive organs are the salivary glands, liver, gallbladder, and pancreas.

<u>Mouth and Stomach</u>

The mouth is the entrance to the digestive system. Here, the mechanical and chemical digestion of the food begins. The food is chewed mechanically by the teeth and shaped into a **bolus** by the tongue so that it can be more easily swallowed by the esophagus. The food also becomes more watery and pliable with the addition of saliva secreted from the salivary glands, the largest of which are the parotid glands. The glands also secrete **amylase** in the saliva, an enzyme which begins chemical digestion and breakdown of the carbohydrates and sugars in the food.

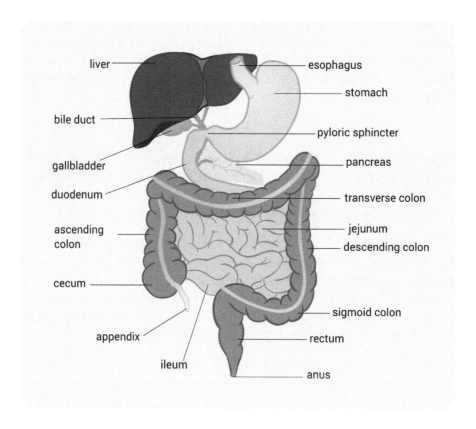

The food then moves through the pharynx and down the muscular esophagus to the stomach.

The stomach is a large, muscular sac-like organ at the distal end of the esophagus. Here, the bolus is subjected to more mechanical and chemical digestion. As it passes through the stomach, it is physically squeezed and crushed while additional secretions turn it into a watery nutrient-filled liquid that exits into the small intestine as **chyme.**

The stomach secretes a great many substances into the **lumen** of the digestive tract. Some cells produce gastrin, a hormone that prompts other cells in the stomach to secrete a gastric acid composed mostly of hydrochloric acid (HCl). The HCl is at such a high concentration and low pH that it denatures most proteins and degrades a lot of organic matter. The stomach also secretes mucous to form a protective film that keeps the corrosive acid from dissolving its own cells. Gaps in this mucous layer can lead to peptic ulcers. Finally, the stomach also uses digestive enzymes like proteases and lipases to break down proteins and fats; although there are some gastric lipases here, the stomach is most known for breaking down proteins.

Small Intestine

The chyme from the stomach enters the first part of the small intestine, the **duodenum,** through the **pyloric sphincter,** and its extreme acidity is partly neutralized by sodium bicarbonate secreted along with mucous. The presence of chyme in the duodenum triggers the secretion of the hormones secretin and cholecystokinin (CCK). Secretin acts on the pancreas to dump more sodium bicarbonate into the small intestine so that the pH is kept at a reasonable level, while CCK acts on the gallbladder to release the **bile** that it has been storing. Bile is a substance produced by the liver and stored in the gallbladder which helps to **emulsify** or dissolve fats and lipids.

Because of the bile which aids in lipid absorption and the secreted lipases which break down fats, the duodenum is the chief site of fat digestion in the body. The duodenum also represents the last major site of chemical digestion in the digestive tract, as the other two sections of the small intestine (the **jejunum** and **ileum**) are instead heavily involved in absorption of nutrients.

The small intestine reaches 40 feet in length, and its cells are arranged in small finger-like projections called **villi.** This is due to its key role in the absorption of nearly all nutrients from the ingested and digested food, effectively transferring them from the lumen of the GI tract to the bloodstream where they travel to the cells which need them. These nutrients include simple sugars like glucose from carbohydrates, amino acids from proteins, emulsified fats, electrolytes like sodium and potassium, minerals like iron and zinc, and vitamins like D and B12. Vitamin B12's absorption, though it takes place in the intestines, is actually aided by **intrinsic factor** that was released into the chyme back in the stomach.

Large Intestine

The leftover parts of food which remain unabsorbed or undigested in the lumen of the small intestine next travel through the **large intestine**, which may also be referred to as the **large bowel** or **colon.** The large intestine is mainly responsible for water absorption. As the chyme at this stage no longer has anything useful that can be absorbed by the body, it is now referred to as **waste,** and it is stored in the large intestine until it can be excreted from the body. Removing the liquid from the waste transforms it from liquid to solid stool, or **feces.**

This waste first passes from the small intestine to the **cecum**, a pouch which forms the first part of the large intestine. In herbivores, it provides a place for bacteria to digest cellulose, but in humans most of it is vestigial and is known as the appendix. From the cecum, waste next travels up the ascending colon, across the transverse colon, down the descending colon, and through the sigmoid colon to the rectum. The rectum is responsible for the final storage of waste before being expelled through the **anus.** The anal canal is a small portion of the rectum leading through to the anus and the outside of the body.

Pancreas

The **pancreas** has endocrine and exocrine functions. The endocrine function involves releasing the hormones insulin, which decreases blood sugar (glucose) levels, and glucagon, which increases blood sugar (glucose) levels, directly into the bloodstream. Both hormones are produced in the **islets of Langerhans,** insulin in the beta cells and glucagon in the alpha cells.

The major part of the gland has exocrine function, which consists of acinar cells secreting inactive digestive enzymes (**zymogens**) into the main pancreatic duct. The main pancreatic duct joins the common bile duct, which empties into the small intestine (specifically the duodenum). The digestive enzymes are then activated and take part in the digestion of carbohydrates, proteins, and fats within chyme (the mixture of partially digested food and digestive juices).

Urinary System

The **urinary system** is made up of the kidneys, ureters, urinary bladder, and the urethra. It is the system responsible for removing waste products and balancing water and electrolyte concentrations in the blood. The urinary system has many important functions related to waste excretion. It regulates the concentrations of sodium, potassium, chloride, calcium, and other ions in the filtrate by controlling the amount of each that is reabsorbed during filtration. The reabsorption or secretion of hydrogen ions and bicarbonate contributes to the maintenance of blood pH. Certain kidney cells can detect any reductions in blood volume and pressure. If that happens, they secrete renin which will activate a hormone that causes increased reabsorption of sodium ions and water, raising volume and pressure. Under hypoxic conditions, kidney cells will secrete erythropoietin in order to stimulate red blood cell production. It also synthesizes **calcitriol**, which is a hormone derivative of vitamin D3 that aids in calcium ion absorption by the intestinal epithelium.

Under normal circumstances, humans have two functioning **kidneys** in the lower back and on either side of the spinal cord. They are the main organs that are responsible for filtering waste products out of the blood and regulating blood water and electrolyte levels. Blood enters the kidney through the renal artery and urea and wastes are removed while water and the acidity/alkalinity of the blood is adjusted. Toxic substances and drugs are also filtered. Blood exits through the renal vein and the urine waste travels through the ureter to the bladder where it is stored until it is eliminated through the urethra.

The kidneys have an outer **renal cortex** and an inner **renal medulla** that contain millions of tiny filtering units called **nephrons.** Nephrons have two parts: a glomerulus, which is the filter, and a tubule. The **glomerulus** is a network of capillaries covered by the **Bowman's capsule**, which is the entrance to the tubule. As blood enters the kidneys via the renal artery, the glomerulus allows for fluid and waste products to pass through it and enter the tubule. Blood cells and large molecules, such as proteins, do not pass through and remain in the blood. The **filtrate** passes through the tubule, which has several parts. The proximal tubule comes first, and then the descending and ascending limbs of the loop of Henle dip into the medulla, followed by the distal tubule and collecting duct. The journey through the tubule involves a balancing act that regulates blood osmolarity, pH, and electrolytes exchange of materials between the tubule and the blood stream. The final product at the collecting tubule is called urine, and it is delivered to the bladder by the ureter. The most central part of the kidney is the **renal pelvis**, and it acts as a funnel by delivering the urine from the millions of the collecting tubules to the **ureters**. The filtered blood exits through the renal vein and is returned to circulation.

Here's a look at the genitourinary system:

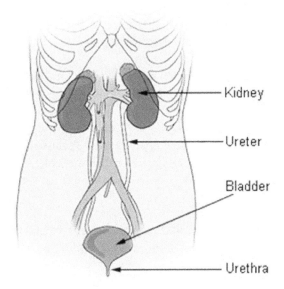

2Here's a close up look at the kidney:

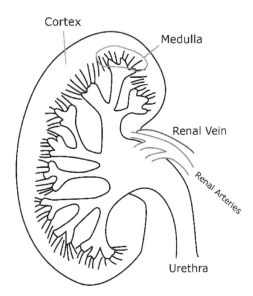

Waste Excretion
Once urine accumulates, it leaves the kidneys. The urine travels through the ureters into the **urinary bladder,** a muscular organ that is hollow and elastic. As more urine enters the urinary bladder, its walls stretch and become thinner so there is no significant difference in internal pressure. The urinary bladder stores the urine until the body is ready for urination, at which time the muscles contract and force the urine through the **urethra** and out of the body.

Reproductive System

The **reproductive system** is responsible for producing, storing, nourishing, and transporting functional reproductive cells, or gametes, in the human body. It includes the reproductive organs, also known as **gonads**, the reproductive tract, the accessory glands and organs that secrete fluids into the reproductive tract, and the **perineal structures**, which are the external genitalia.

Reproduction involves the passing of genes from one generation to the next, and that is accomplished through haploid gametes. Gametes have gone through meiosis and have 23 chromosomes, half the normal number. The male gamete is **sperm**, and the female gamete is an **egg** or **ovum.** When a sperm fertilizes an egg, they create a **zygote,** which is the first cell of a new organism. The zygote has a full set of 46 chromosomes because it received 23 from each parent. Because of sperm and egg development gene shuffling, sperm and egg chromosome sets are all different which results in the variety seen in humans.

Male Reproductive System

The entire male reproductive system is designed to generate sperm and produce semen that facilitate fertilization of eggs, the female gametes. The testes are the endocrine glands that secrete **testosterone**, a hormone that is important for secondary sex characteristics and sperm development, or **spermatogenesis**. Testosterone is in the androgen steroid-hormone family. The testes also produce and store 500 million spermatocytes, which are the male gametes, each day. Testes are housed in the **scrotum,** which is a sac that hangs outside the body so that spermatogenesis occurs at cooler and optimal conditions.

The **seminiferous tubules** within the testes produce sperm and then they travel to **epididymis** where they are stored as they mature. Then, the sperm move to the **ejaculatory duct** via the **vas deference**. The ejaculatory duct contains more than just sperm. The **seminal vesicles** secrete an alkaline substance that will help sperm survive in the acidic vagina. The prostate gland secretes enzymes bathed in a milky white fluid that is important for thinning semen after ejaculation to increase its likelihood of reaching the egg. The **bulbourethral,** or **Cowper's, gland** secretes an alkaline fluid that lubricates the urethra prior to ejaculation to neutralize any acidic urine residue.

The sperm, along with all the exocrine secretions, are collectively called **semen.** Their destination is the vagina and they can only get there if the penis is erect due to arousal and increased circulation. During sexual intercourse, ejaculation will forcefully expel the contents of the semen and effectively deliver the sperm to the egg. The muscular prostate gland is important for ejaculation. Each ejaculation releases 2 to 6 million sperm. Sperm has a whip-like flagellum tail that facilitates movement.

Female Reproductive System

The **vagina** is the passageway that sperm must travel through to reach an egg, the female gamete. Surrounding the vagina are the labia minor and labia major, both of which are folds that protect the urethra and the vaginal opening. The **clitoris** is rich in nerve-endings, making it sensitive and highly stimulated during sexual intercourse. It is above the vagina and urethra. An exocrine gland called the **Bartholin's glands** secretes a fluid during arousal that is important for lubrication.

The female gonads are the **ovaries.** Ovaries generally produce one immature gamete, an egg or oocyte, per month. They are also responsible for secreting the hormones **estrogen** and **progesterone**. Fertilization cannot happen unless the ejaculated sperm finds the egg, which are only available at certain times of the month. Eggs, or ova, develop in the ovaries in clusters surrounded by follicles, and after puberty, they are delivered to the uterus once a month via the **Fallopian tubes**. The 28-day average journey of the egg to the uterus is called the menstrual cycle and it is highly regulated by the endocrine system. The regulatory hormones Gonadotropin releasing hormone (GnRH), luteinizing hormone (LH), and follicle-stimulating hormone (FSH) orchestrate the menstrual cycle. Ovarian hormones estrogen and progesterone are also important in timing as well as for vascularization of the uterus in preparation for pregnancy. **Fertilization** usually happens around ovulation, which is when the egg is inside the Fallopian tube. The resulting zygote travels down the tube and implants into the uterine wall. The uterus protects and nourishes the developing embryo for nine months until it is ready for the outside environment.

If the egg released is unfertilized, the uterine lining will slough off during **menstruation.** Should a fertilized egg, called a **zygote**, reach the uterus, it will embed itself into the uterine wall due to uterine vascularization that will deliver blood, nutrients, and antibodies to the developing embryo. The uterus is where the embryo will develop for the next nine months. **Mammary glands** are important female reproductive structures because they produce milk they provide for their young during **lactation**. Milk contains nutrients and antibodies that benefit the baby.

Practice Questions

1. Why do arteries have valves?
    a. They have valves to maintain high blood pressure so that capillaries diffuse nutrients properly.
    b. Their valves are designed to prevent backflow due to their low blood pressure.
    c. The valves have no known purpose and thus appear to be unnecessary.
    d. They do not have valves, but veins do.

2. Which locations in the digestive system are sites of chemical digestion?
    I. Mouth
    II. Stomach
    III. Small Intestine

    a. II only
    b. III only
    c. II and III only
    d. I, II, and III

3. Which of the following are functions of the urinary system?
    I. Synthesizing calcitriol and secreting erythropoietin
    II. Regulating the concentrations of sodium, potassium, chloride, calcium, and other ions
    III. Reabsorbing or secreting hydrogen ions and bicarbonate
    IV. Detecting reductions in blood volume and pressure

    a. I, II, and III
    b. II and III
    c. II, III, and IV
    d. All of the above

4. If the pressure in the pulmonary artery is increased above normal, which chamber of the heart will be affected first?
    a. The right atrium
    b. The left atrium
    c. The right ventricle
    d. The left ventricle

5. What is the purpose of sodium bicarbonate when released into the lumen of the small intestine?
    a. It works to chemically digest fats in the chyme.
    b. It decreases the pH of the chyme so as to prevent harm to the intestine.
    c. It works to chemically digest proteins in the chyme.
    d. It increases the pH of the chyme so as to prevent harm to the intestine.

6. Which of the following describes a reflex arc?
    a. The storage and recall of memory
    b. The maintenance of visual and auditory acuity
    c. The autoregulation of heart rate and blood pressure
    d. A stimulus and response controlled by the spinal cord

7. Ligaments connect what?
   a. Muscle to muscle
   b. Bone to bone
   c. Bone to muscle
   d. Muscle to tendon

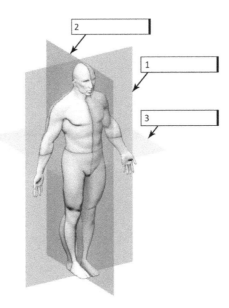

8. Identify the correct sequence of the 3 primary body planes as numbered 1, 2, and 3 in the above image.
   a. Plane 1 is coronal, plane 2 is sagittal, and plane 3 is transverse.
   b. Plane 1 is sagittal, plane 2 is coronal, and plane 3 is medial.
   c. Plane 1 is coronal, plane 2 is sagittal, and plane 3 is medial.
   d. Plane 1 is sagittal, plane 2 is coronal, and plane 3 is transverse.

9. Which of the following is NOT a major function of the respiratory system in humans?
   a. It provides a large surface area for gas exchange of oxygen and carbon dioxide.
   b. It helps regulate the blood's pH.
   c. It helps cushion the heart against jarring motions.
   d. It is responsible for vocalization.

10. Which of the following is NOT a function of the forebrain?
   a. To regulate blood pressure and heart rate
   b. To perceive and interpret emotional responses like fear and anger
   c. To perceive and interpret visual input from the eyes
   d. To integrate voluntary movement

11. A patient's body is not properly filtering blood. Which of the following body parts is most likely malfunctioning?
   a. Medulla
   B. Heart
   C. Nephrons
   D. Renal cortex

12. A pediatrician notes that an infant's cartilage is disappearing and being replaced by bone. What process has the doctor observed?
    a. Mineralization
    b. Ossification
    c. Osteoporosis
    d. Calcification

13. Which of the following creates sperm?
    a. Prostate gland
    b. Seminal vesicles
    c. Scrotum
    d. Seminiferous tubules

14. Which of the following functions corresponds to the parasympathetic nervous system?
    a. It stimulates the fight-or-flight response.
    b. It increases heart rate.
    c. It stimulates digestion.
    d. It increases bronchiole dilation.

15. Which of the following is the gland that helps regulate calcium levels?
    a. Osteotoid gland
    b. Pineal gland
    c. Parathyroid glands
    d. Thymus gland

16. What makes bone resistant to shattering?
    a. The calcium salts deposited in the bone
    b. The collagen fibers
    c. The bone marrow and network of blood vessels
    d. The intricate balance of minerals and collagen fibers

17. What type of vessel carries oxygen-rich blood from the heart to other tissues of the body?
    a. Veins
    b. Intestines
    c. Bronchioles
    d. Arteries

18. The somatic nervous system is responsible for which of the following?
    a. Breathing
    b. Thought
    c. Movement
    d. Fear

19. Which blood component is chiefly responsible for clotting?
    a. Platelets
    b. Red blood cells
    c. Antigens
    d. Plasma cells

20. What is the function of the sinuses?
    a. To trap the many airborne pathogens
    b. To direct air down the trachea rather than the esophagus
    c. To warm, humidify, and filter air
    d. To sweep away pathogens and direct them toward the top of the trachea

21. Which of the following structures acts like a funnel by delivering the urine from the millions of the collecting tubules to the ureters?
    a. The renal pelvis
    b. The renal cortex
    c. The renal medulla
    d. Bowman's capsule

22. A cluster of capillaries that functions as the main filter of the blood entering the kidney is known as which of the following?
    a. The Bowman's capsule
    b. The Loop of Henle
    c. The glomerulus
    d. The nephron

23. What is the name for the sac-shaped structures in which carbon dioxide and oxygen exchange takes place?
    a. Kidneys
    b. Medulla oblongata
    c. Alveoli
    d. Bronchioles

24. The muscular tube that connects the outer surface to the cervix in a woman's birth canal is referred to as which of the following?
    a. The uterus
    b. The cervix
    c. The vagina
    d. The ovaries

25. Which of the following organs functions both as an endocrine and exocrine gland?
    a. The kidney
    b. The spleen
    c. The pancreas
    d. The stomach

Answer Explanations

1. D: Veins have valves, but arteries do not. Valves in veins are designed to prevent backflow, since they are the furthest blood vessels from the pumping action of the heart and steadily increase in volume (which decreases the available pressure). Capillaries diffuse nutrients properly because of their thin walls and high surface area and are not particularly dependent on positive pressure.

2. D: Mechanical digestion is physical digestion of food and tearing it into smaller pieces using force. This occurs in the stomach and mouth. Chemical digestion involves chemically changing the food and breaking it down into small organic compounds that can be utilized by the cell to build molecules. The salivary glands in the mouth secrete amylase that breaks down starch, which begins chemical digestion. The stomach contains enzymes such as pepsinogen/pepsin and gastric lipase, which chemically digest protein and fats, respectively. The small intestine continues to digest protein using the enzymes trypsin and chymotrypsin. It also digests fats with the help of bile from the liver and lipase from the pancreas. These organs act as exocrine glands because they secrete substances through a duct. Carbohydrates are digested in the small intestine with the help of pancreatic amylase, gut bacterial flora and fauna, and brush border enzymes like lactose. Brush border enzymes are contained in the towel-like microvilli in the small intestine that soak up nutrients.

3. D: The urinary system has many functions, the primary of which is removing waste products and balancing water and electrolyte concentrations in the blood. It also plays a key role in regulating ion concentrations, such as sodium, potassium, chloride, and calcium, in the filtrate. The urinary system helps maintain blood pH by reabsorbing or secreting hydrogen ions and bicarbonate as necessary. Certain kidney cells can detect reductions in blood volume and pressure and then can secrete renin to activate a hormone that causes increased reabsorption of sodium ions and water. This serves to raise blood volume and pressure. Kidney cells secrete erythropoietin under hypoxic conditions to stimulate red blood cell production. They also synthesize calcitriol, a hormone derivative of vitamin D3, which aids in calcium ion absorption by the intestinal epithelium.

4. C: The blood leaves the right ventricle through a semi-lunar valve and goes through the pulmonary artery to the lungs. Any increase in pressure in the artery will eventually affect the contractibility of the right ventricle. Blood enters the right atrium from the superior and inferior venae cava veins, and blood leaves the right atrium through the tricuspid valve to the right ventricle. Blood enters the left atrium from the pulmonary veins carrying oxygenated blood from the lungs. Blood flows from the left atrium to the left ventricle through the mitral valve and leaves the left ventricle through a semi-lunar valve to enter the aorta.

5. D: Sodium bicarbonate, a very effective base, has the chief function to increase the pH of the chyme. Chyme leaving the stomach has a very low pH, due to the high amounts of acid that are used to digest and break down food. If this is not neutralized, the walls of the small intestine will be damaged and may form ulcers. Sodium bicarb is produced by the pancreas and released in response to pyloric stimulation so that it can neutralize the acid. It has little to no digestive effect.

6. D: A reflex arc is a simple nerve pathway involving a stimulus, a synapse, and a response that is controlled by the spinal cord—not the brain. The knee-jerk reflex is an example of a reflex arc. The stimulus is the hammer touching the tendon, reaching the synapse in the spinal cord by an afferent pathway. The response is the resulting muscle contraction reaching the muscle by an efferent pathway. None of the remaining processes is a simple reflex. Memories are processed and stored in the hippocampus in the limbic system. The visual center is located in the occipital lobe, while auditory processing occurs in the temporal lobe. The sympathetic and parasympathetic divisions of the autonomic nervous system control heart and blood pressure.

7. B: Ligaments connect bone to bone. Tendons connect muscle to bone. Both are made of dense, fibrous connective tissue (primary Type 1 collagen) to give strength. However, tendons are more organized, especially in the long axis direction like muscle fibers themselves, and they have more collagen. This arrangement makes more sense because muscles have specific orientations of their fibers, so they contract in somewhat predictable directions. Ligaments are less organized and more of a woven pattern because bone connections are not as organized as bundles or muscle fibers, so ligaments must have strength in multiple directions to protect against injury.

8. A: The three primary body planes are coronal, sagittal, and transverse. The coronal or frontal plane, named for the plane in which a corona or halo might appear in old paintings, divides the body vertically into front and back sections. The sagittal plane, named for the path an arrow might take when shot at the body, divides the body vertically into right and left sections. The transverse plane divides the body horizontally into upper or superior and lower or inferior sections. There is no medial plane, per se. The anatomical direction medial simply references a location close or closer to the center of the body than another location.

9. C: Although the lungs may provide some cushioning for the heart when the body is violently struck, this is not a major function of the respiratory system. Its most notable function is that of gas exchange for oxygen and carbon dioxide, but it also plays a vital role in the regulation of blood pH. The aqueous form of carbon dioxide, carbonic acid, is a major pH buffer of the blood, and the respiratory system directly controls how much carbon dioxide stays and is released from the blood through respiration. The respiratory system also enables vocalization and forms the basis for the mode of speech and language used by most humans.

10. A: The forebrain contains the cerebrum, the thalamus, the hypothalamus, and the limbic system. The limbic system is chiefly responsible for the perception of emotions through the amygdale, while the cerebrum interprets sensory input and generates movement. Specifically, the occipital lobe receives visual input, and the primary motor cortex in the frontal lobe is the controller of voluntary movement. The hindbrain, specifically the medulla oblongata and brain stem, control and regulate blood pressure and heart rate.

11. C: Nephrons are responsible for filtering blood. When functioning properly they allow blood cells and nutrients to go back into the bloodstream while sending waste to the bladder. However, nephrons can fail at doing this, particularly when blood flood to the kidneys is limited. The medulla (also called the renal medulla) (*A*) and the renal cortex (*D*) are both parts of the kidney but are not specifically responsible for filtering blood. The medulla is in the inner part of the kidney and contains the nephrons. The renal cortex is the outer part of the kidney. The heart (*B*) is responsible for pumping blood throughout the body rather than filtering it.

12. B: Ossification is the process by which cartilage, a soft, flexible substance is replaced by bone throughout the body. All humans regardless of age have cartilage, but cartilage in some areas goes away to make way for bones.

13. D: The seminiferous tubules are responsible for sperm production. Had *testicles* been an answer choice, it would also have been correct since it houses the seminiferous tubules. The prostate gland (*A*) secretes enzymes that help nourish sperm after creation. The seminal vesicles (*B*) secrete some of the components of semen. The scrotum (*C*) is the pouch holding the testicles.

14. C: The parasympathetic nervous system is related to calm, peaceful times without stress that require no immediate decisions. It relaxes the fight-or-flight response, slows heart rate to a comfortable pace, and decreases bronchiole dilation to a normal size. The sympathetic nervous system, on the other hand, is in charge of the fight-or-flight response and works to increase blood pressure and oxygen absorption.

15. C: The parathryroid gland impacts calcium levels by secreting parathyroid hormone (PTH). Osteotoid gland is not a real gland. The pineal gland regulates sleep by secreting melatonin, and the thymus gland focuses on immunity. *Thyroid* would also be a correct answer choice as it influences the levels of circulating calcium.

16. D: Bony matrix is an intricate lattice of collagen fibers and mineral salts, particularly calcium and phosphorus. The mineral salts are strong but brittle, and the collagen fibers are weak but flexible, so the combination of the two makes bone resistant to shattering and able to withstand the normal forces applied to it.

17. D: Arteries carry oxygen-rich blood from the heart to the other tissues of the body. Veins carry oxygen-poor blood back to the heart. Intestines carry digested food through the body. Bronchioles are passageways that carry air from the nose and mouth to the lungs.

18. C: The somatic nervous system is the voluntary nervous system, responsible for voluntary movement. It includes nerves that transmit signals from the brain to the muscles of the body. Breathing is controlled by the autonomic nervous system. Thought and fear are complex processes that occur in the brain, which is part of the central nervous system.

19. A: Platelets are the blood components responsible for clotting. There are between 150,000 and 450,000 platelets in healthy blood. When a clot forms, platelets adhere to the injured area of the vessel and promote a molecular cascade that results in adherence of more platelets. Ultimately, the platelet aggregation results in recruitment of a protein called fibrin, which adds structure to the clot. Too many platelets can cause clotting disorders. Not enough leads to bleeding disorders.

20. C: The sinuses function to warm, filter, and humidify air that is inhaled. Choice *A* is incorrect because mucus traps airborne pathogens. Choice *B* is incorrect because the epiglottis is the structure in the pharynx that covers the trachea during swallowing to prevent food from entering it. Lastly, Choice *D*, sweeping away pathogens and directing them toward the top of the trachea, is the function of cilia. Respiratory structures, such as the nasal passages and trachea, are lined with mucus and cilia.

21. A: The renal pelvis acts like a funnel by delivering the urine from the millions of the collecting tubules to the ureters. It is the most central part of the kidney. The renal cortex is the outer layer of the kidney, while the renal medulla is the inner layer. The renal medulla contains the functional units of the kidneys—nephrons—which function to filter the blood. Choice *D*, Bowman's capsule, is the name for the structure that covers the glomeruli.

22. C: A cluster of capillaries that functions as the main filter of the blood entering the kidney is known as the glomerulus, so Choice *C* is correct. The Bowman's capsule surrounds the glomerulus and receives fluid and solutes from it; therefore, Choice *A* is incorrect. The loop of Henle is a part of the kidney tubule where water and nutrients are reabsorbed, so *B* is false. The nephron is the unit containing all of these anatomical features, making Choice *D* incorrect as well.

23. C: The alveoli are small sac-shaped structures at the end of the bronchioles where gas exchange takes place. The bronchioles are tubes through which air travels. The kidneys and medulla oblongata do not directly affect oxygen and carbon dioxide exchange.

24. C: The uterus and ovaries aren't part of the birth canal, so Choices *A* and *D* are false. The cervix is the uppermost portion of the birth canal, so Choice *B* is incorrect, making Choice *C* the correct answer, as the vagina is the muscular tube on the lowermost portion of the birth canal that connects the exterior environment to the cervix.

25. C: The pancreas functions as an exocrine gland because it secretes enzymes that break down food components. It also functions as an endocrine gland because it secretes hormones that regulate blood sugar levels. The kidney isn't a gland; it is an organ located directly below the adrenal glands. The stomach is an exocrine gland because it secretes hydrochloric acid. Like the kidney, the spleen is an organ, not a gland. Therefore, the only correct answer is *C*.

Physics

Nature of Motion

People have been studying the movement of objects since ancient times, sometimes prompted by curiosity, and sometimes by necessity. On Earth, items move according to specific guidelines and have motion that is fairly predictable. The measurement of an object's movement or change in position (x), over a change in time (t) is an object's **speed.** The **average speed** of an object is defined as the distance that the object travels divided by how long it takes the object to travel that distance. When the direction is included with the speed, it is referred to as the **velocity**. A "change in position" refers to the difference in location of an object's starting point and an object's ending point. In science, this change is represented by the Greek letter Delta, Δ.

$$velocity\ (v) = \frac{\Delta x}{\Delta t}$$

Distance is measured in meters, and time is measured in seconds. The standard scientific units for speed and velocity are meters/second (m/s), but units of miles/hour (mph) are also commonly used in America.

$$\frac{meters}{second} = \frac{m}{s}$$

Average velocity is calculated by averaging the beginning or initial velocity and the ending or final velocity of an object.

If a measurement includes its direction, it is called a **vector quantity**; otherwise, the measurement is called a **scalar quantity** and has only a numeric value without a particular direction. For example, speed is a scalar quantity while velocity is a vector quantity.

Acceleration

While an object's speed measures how fast the object's position will change in a certain amount of time, an object's **acceleration** measures how fast the object's speed will change in a certain amount of time. Acceleration can be thought of as the change in velocity or speed (Δv) divided by the change in the time (Δt).

$$acceleration\ (a) = \frac{\Delta v}{\Delta t}$$

Velocity is measured in meters/second and time is measured in seconds, so the standard unit for acceleration is meters / second2 (m/s2).

$$\frac{meters/second}{second} = \frac{meters}{second^2} = \frac{m}{s^2}$$

Acceleration is expressed by using both magnitude and direction, so it is a vector quantity like velocity. Acceleration is present when an object is slowing down, speeding up, or changing direction, since these represent instances where velocity is changing. This means that forces like friction and gravity accelerate objects and increase or decrease their velocities over time.

Projectile Motion

Projectile motion describes the way in which a projectile will move when the only force acting upon it is gravity. Since the force of Earth's gravity is nearly constant at sea level, its magnitude is approximated as a rate of 9.8 m/s2. For projectile motion problems, the projectile is assumed to travel a curved path to the ground and ignore air resistance, wind speed, and other such complications.

Projectile motion has two components: horizontal and vertical. Without air resistance, there is no horizontal acceleration, so the horizontal velocity won't change. However, the vertical velocity will change because of gravity's acceleration on the projectile. A sample parabolic curve of projectile motion is shown below.

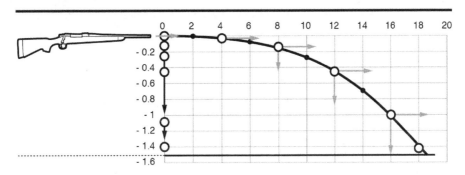

Horizontal distance (d_x) is defined as the relationship between velocity (v_x) and time (t), where x is the movement along the horizontal plane (x-axis).

$$d_x = v_x t$$

Because of the force of gravity, the vertical velocity and position is continuously changing and thus more complicated to calculate. The following equations are different expressions of vertical motion:

$$v_f{}^2 = v_i{}^2 + 2ad$$

$$d = \frac{1}{2}at^2 + v_i t$$

$$v_f = v_i + at$$

These equations use v_f as the final velocity, v_i as the initial velocity, a as the acceleration, d as the horizontal distance traveled, and t as the time to describe functions of motion.

Newton's Laws of Motion

Sir Isaac Newton spent a great deal of time studying objects, forces, and how an object's motion responds to forces. Newton made great advancements by using mathematics to describe the motion of objects and to predict future motions of objects by applying his mathematical models to situations.

Through his extensive research, Newton is credited for summarizing the basic laws of motion for objects here on Earth. These laws are as follows:

1. The law of inertia: An object in motion will remain in motion, unless acted upon by an outside force. An object at rest remains at rest, unless acted upon by an outside force. Simply put, **inertia** is the natural tendency of an object to continue along with what it is already doing; an outside force would have to act upon the object to make it change its course. This includes an object that is sitting still.

2. F = ma: The **force (F)** on an object is equal to the mass (m) multiplied by the acceleration (a) on that object. **Mass (m)** refers to the amount of a substance while acceleration (a) refers to a change in velocity over time.

- In the case of a projectile falling to Earth's surface, the acceleration is due to gravity.

- Multiplying an object's mass by its gravitational acceleration gives the special force that is called the object's **weight (W).** Note that weight is a force and is a vector quantity while mass is in kilograms and is a scalar quantity, as it has no acceleration.

- Forces are typically measured in **Newtons** (N), which are a derived SI unit equal to $1 \frac{kg \cdot m}{s^2}$. You can find an object's weight in Newtons by multiplying its mass (in kilograms) by the acceleration of gravity (9.8 m/s2 for Earth).

3. For every action, there is an equal and opposite reaction. This means that, if a book drops onto a desk, the book will exert a force on the desk due to hitting it, but the desk will also exert an equal force on the book in the opposite direction. This is what sometimes causes fallen objects to bounce once or twice after hitting the ground.

A clear understanding of force is crucial to using Newton's laws of motion. **Forces** are anything acting upon an object either in motion or at rest; this includes friction and gravity. These forces can push or pull on a mass, and they have a magnitude and a direction. Forces are represented by a **vector,** which is the arrow lined up along the direction of the force with its tip at the point of application. The magnitude of the force is represented by the length of the vector: Large forces have long vector lengths.

Friction

Friction is a resistance to movement that always imparts a negative acceleration to an object. Because it accelerates an object in the opposite direction than it wants to go, friction will cause moving objects to slow down and eventually stop. Frictional force depends on several factors including the texture of the two surfaces and the amount of contact force pushing the surfaces together. There are four types of friction: static, sliding, rolling, and fluid friction. **Static friction** occurs between stationary objects, while **sliding friction** occurs when solid objects slide over each other. **Rolling friction** happens when a solid object rolls over another solid object, and **fluid friction** is a friction caused by an object moving through a fluid or through fluid layers. These 'fluids' can be either a gas or a liquid, so this also includes air resistance.

Rotation

Rotating and spinning objects have a special type of movement. A spinning top can move across a table, demonstrating linear motion, but it can also spin in place, demonstrating angular motion. Just as a car moves from place to place by changing its location, its velocity, and its acceleration, so too can a rotating object change its orientation, its angular velocity, and its angular acceleration.

For linear movement, the first thing that is described is the object's displacement. The **displacement** of the object is how far it moves from its starting location; this linear change in location is usually represented by the symbol Δx. However, for the angular movement of a simple solid like a sphere, the distance that its surface travels isn't a good measure of its angular movement, since a large sphere would have to rotate a much smaller degree to move the same distance as a small sphere would. This angular distance is referred to as S, or the arc length.

A better measure of angular movement is the **angular displacement θ,** which is defined as the angle through which the object will rotate. Because there are a standard 360° in all circles, angular displacement can be used to compare angular movement between objects of different sizes, making it a much more versatile tool than the arc length. However, although a circle can be split up into 360 degrees, it can also be visualized as being split up into 2π **radians,** where radians is a unit similar to degrees that describes angles. The 2π is usually used in physics because a circle's circumference has a value of 2π times its radius, and radians is an easier unit to use than is degrees.

The angular displacement can be found by dividing the arc length that an object rotates through by the radius of the object's rotation. For example, if an object completes 1 full rotation, it has rotated through 360°. It has also traveled an arc length equal to its circumference, or $2\pi r$. Plugging this arc length S into the equation below, it can be seen that the angular displacement is 2π, which is correct since it is equal to the 360° as discussed previously.

$$angular\ displacement\ (\theta) = \frac{S}{r}$$

The angular speed or **angular velocity, w,** is the measure of how quickly the object is rotating, and w is defined as the angular displacement that is accomplished in a certain amount of time, as shown below.

$$angular\ speed\ (\omega) = \frac{\Delta\theta}{\Delta t}$$

Similar to linear velocity, angular velocity may accelerate due to external forces, and this angular acceleration is given by the variable α. Its equation, the change in angular velocity over a change in time, is given below.

$$angular\ acceleration\ (\alpha) = \frac{\Delta\omega}{\Delta t}$$

When objects are exhibiting circular motion, they also demonstrate the **conservation of angular momentum,** meaning that the angular momentum of a system is always constant, regardless of the placement of the mass. **Rotational inertia** can be affected by how far the mass of the object is placed with respect to the center of rotation (**axis of rotation**). The larger the distance between the mass and the center of rotation, the slower the rotational velocity. Conversely, if the mass is closer to the center of rotation, the rotational velocity increases. A change in one affects the other, thus conserving the angular momentum. This holds true if no external forces act upon the system.

Circular Motion

Circular motion is similar in many ways to linear (straight line) motion; however, there are a few additional points to note. In uniform circular motion, a spinning object is always linearly accelerating because it is always changing direction. The force causing this constant acceleration on or around an axis is called the **centripetal force,** and it is often associated with centripetal acceleration. Centripetal force always pulls toward the axis of rotation; this means that the force will always pull towards the center of the rotation circle. The relationship between the velocity (v) of an object and the radius (r) of the circle is **centripetal acceleration**, and the equation is as follows:

$$centripetal\ acceleration\ (a_c) = \frac{v^2}{r}$$

According to Newton's law, force is the combination of two factors, mass and acceleration. This is demonstrated by centripetal force. Centripetal force is shown mathematically by using the mass of an object (m), the velocity (v), and the radius (r).

$$centripetal\ force\ (F_c) = \frac{mv^2}{r}$$

Kinetic and Potential Energy

The two primary forms of energy are kinetic energy and potential energy. **Kinetic energy**, or KE, involves the energy of motion, and is easily found for Newtonian physics by an object's mass in kilograms and velocity in meters per second. Kinetic energy can be calculated using the following equation:

$$KE = \frac{1}{2}mv^2$$

Potential energy represents the energy possessed by an object by virtue of its position. In the classical example, an object's gravitational potential energy can be found as a simple function of its height or by what distance it drops. Potential energy, or PE, may be calculated using the following equation:

$$PE = mgh$$

Both kinetic energy and potential energy are scalar quantities measured in **Joules**. One Joule is the amount of energy that can push an object with 1 Newton of force for 1 meter, so it is also referred to as a Newton-meter. As mentioned previously, the **Law of Conservation of Energy** states that energy can neither be created nor destroyed. Therefore, potential and kinetic energy can be transformed into one another, depending on an object's speed and position.

Linear Momentum and Impulse

Motion creates something called **momentum.** This is a calculation of an object's mass multiplied by its velocity. Momentum can be described as the amount an object wants to continue moving along its current course. Momentum in a straight line is called linear momentum. Just as energy can be transferred and conserved, so too can momentum.

Changing the expression of Newton's second law of motion yields a new expression.

$$Force(F) = ma = m \times \frac{\Delta v}{\Delta t}$$

If both sides of the expression are multiplied by the change in time, the law produces the impulse equation.

$$F\Delta t = m\Delta v$$

This equation shows that the amount of force during a length of time creates an **impulse.** This means that if a force acts on an object during a given amount of time, it will have a determined impulse. However, if the same change in velocity happens over a longer amount of time, the required force is much smaller, due to the conservation of momentum.

$$p = mv$$

Linear momentum, p, is found by multiplying the mass of an object by its velocity. Since momentum, like mass and energy, is conserved, Newton's 2nd law can be restated for multiple objects. In this form, it can be used to understand the energy of objects that have interacted, since the conservation of momentum implies that the momentum before and after an interaction must be the same. This is best demonstrated in the case of elastic collision, where an object of mass m_1 with velocity v_1 collides with an object of mass m_2 with velocity v_2 and both object end with velocities v_1' and v_2', respectively.

$$m_1 v_1' + m_2 v_2' = m_1 v_1 + m_2 v_2$$

Universal Gravitation

Newton's **law of universal gravitation** addresses the universality of gravity. Gravity acts as a force at a distance and causes all bodies in the universe to attract each other.

The **force of gravity (F_g)** is proportional to the masses of two objects (m_1 and m_2) and inversely proportional to the square of the distance (r^2) between them. (G is the proportionality constant). This is shown in the following equation:

$$F_g = G \frac{m_1 m_2}{r^2}$$

All objects falling within the Earth's atmosphere are all affected by the force of gravity, so their rates of acceleration will be equal to 9.8 m/s^2, or gravity. Therefore, if two objects are dropped from the same height at the same time, they should hit the ground at the same time. This is irrespective of mass, since the previous kinetics equations don't include mass, so a bowling ball and a feather would theoretically fall at identical rates. Unfortunately, in the Earth's atmosphere, air resistance would slow the feather much more than the bowling ball, so the bowling ball would fall faster, but this effect can be minimized in a vacuum. In other words, without air resistance or other external forces acting on the objects, gravity will affect every object on the Earth with the same rate of acceleration.

Waves and Sound

Waves are periodic disturbances in a gas, liquid, or solid that are created as energy is transmitted. Each part of a wave has a different name and is used in different calculations. The four parts of a wave are the crest, the trough, the amplitude, and the wavelength. The **crest** is the highest point, while the **trough** is the lowest. The **amplitude** is the distance between a peak and the average of the wave; it is also the distance between a trough and the average of the wave, but an amplitude is always positive, since it is an absolute value. Finally, the distance between one wave and the exact same place on the next wave is the **wavelength.**

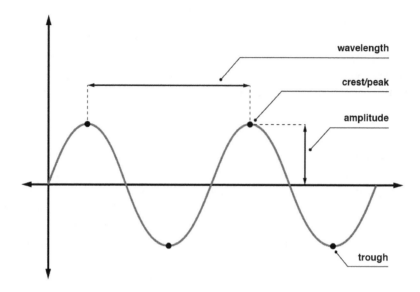

With amplitude and wavelength, it is possible to describe any wave, but an important question still remains unanswered: How fast is the wave traveling? A wave's speed can be shown as either its period or its frequency. A wave's period, T, is how long it takes for the wave to travel one wavelength, while a wave's frequency, f, is how many wavelengths are traveled in one second. These are inversely related, so they are reciprocals of each other, as shown below.

$$f = \frac{1}{T} \text{ and } T = \frac{1}{f}$$

The largest categories of waves are electromagnetic waves and mechanical waves. **Electromagnetic waves** can transmit energy through a vacuum and do not need a medium to travel through, examples of which are light, radio, microwaves, gamma rays, and other forms of electromagnetism. **Mechanical waves** can only transmit energy through another form of matter called a medium. The particles of the medium are shifted as the wave moves through the medium, and can be anything from solids to liquids to gasses. Examples of mechanical waves include auditory sounds heard by human ears in the air as well as percussive shocks like earthquakes.

There are two different forms of waves: transverse and longitudinal waves. **Transverse** waves are waves in which particles of the medium move in a direction perpendicular to the direction waves move, as in most electromagnetic waves. **Compression,** or **longitudinal,** waves are waves in which the particles of the medium move in a direction parallel to the direction the waves move, as in most mechanical waves. A good example of a longitudinal wave is sound. Waves travel within a medium at a speed that is determined by the wavelength (λ) and frequency (f) of the wave.

$$v = f\lambda$$

There is a proportional relationship between the amplitude of a wave and the potential energy in the wave. This means the taller the wave, the more stored energy it is transmitting.

244

Light

Light is an electromagnetic wave that is created by electric and magnetic interactions. Like other electromagnetic waves, light does not need a medium to travel. Light energy can be absorbed and changed into heat, reflected, or even transmitted.

A wave is reflected when it collides with a surface and bounces off, unharmed. The **law of reflection** shows that an **incident ray** (the wave that hits the surface) will bounce off the surface and become a reflected ray (the wave that leaves the surface). Because the wave doesn't lose any energy, the angle at which it hits the surface will be identical to the angle at which it leaves the surface, so the interaction produces identical waves. This is the definition of **reflection**.

On the other hand, a wave is refracted when a wave collides with a surface and bends, such as when the medium it is traveling through changes. Examples of **refraction** include the bending of light as it passes through a prism and sunlight passing through raindrops to create a rainbow.

To understand refraction, a 'normal' line is drawn perpendicular to the surface that the wave will hit. The angle created between the normal line and the incident ray is the angle of incidence, while the angle of reflection is the opposite and equal angle formed between the normal line and the reflected ray. The refraction of light depends on the varying speeds and densities of different media. As light passes through different media, the wave will bend toward or away from the normal line, depending on the material it is transitioning to. **Snell's law** describes this behavior mathematically in the equation that follows:

$$n_1 \sin \theta_1 = n_2 \sin \theta_2$$

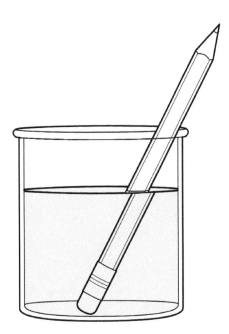

In this equation, n is the index of refraction and θ is the angle of refraction. The **index of refraction** determines the amount of light that bends or refracts when it encounters a medium. Materials that interact with and change the wave more will have higher indices of refraction, and any material's index of refraction can be found by the following equation.

$$n = \frac{c}{v_s}$$

Because the speed of light in a vacuum, c, is constant, it can be used to show how much a material will interact with a wave. The **refractive index, n,** shows how much the speed of light is changed when it travels through the material at a new velocity of v_s.

Optics

Spherical mirrors change the way light reflects. Lenses and curved mirrors are made to focus light in certain ways. There are several terms used to describe and define mirrors and lenses. The **principal axis** is a reference line that usually passes through the center of the curve of the mirror or lens. The **vertex, V,** is the point where the mirror is crossed by the principal axis. The sphere which contains the curve of the mirror has a center called the **center of curvature (C)**. The **focal point (F)** is halfway between the center of curvature and the vertex. The **focal length (f)** is measured by how far the focal point is from the mirror. The following graphic shows a visual representation of these terms in a concave mirror.

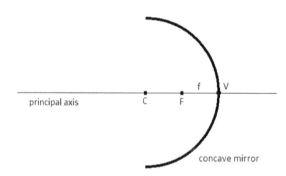

The focal lengths of concave mirrors are positive. Concave mirrors can produce images of various shapes and sizes as well as of different orientations based on the focal length of the mirror and the placement of the object. Convex mirrors differ from concave mirrors in that they have negative focal lengths. The other main difference is that convex mirrors always form images that are reduced in size and upright.

Lenses are pieces of transparent material molded to refract light rays to create an image. There are two types of lenses. Convex lenses, also called **converging lenses**, have positive focal lengths. Concave lenses, or **diverging lenses**, conversely have negative focal lengths. Images in convex lenses can look different depending on the focal length of the lens and where the object is located. Concave lenses only create images that are upright and smaller in size than the object.

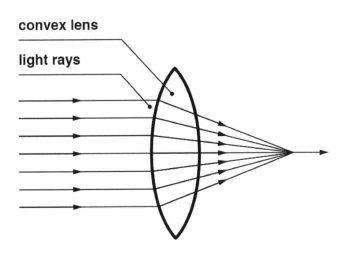

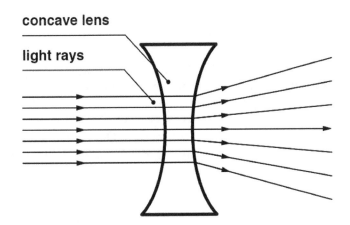

Atomic Structure

All known matter is made of atoms. Atoms have a nucleus composed of **protons** (with a positive charge) and **neutrons** (with no net charge), which is surrounded by a cloud of **electrons** (with negative charges). Since protons have a positive charge and neutrons have a neutral charge, an atom's nucleus typically has an overall positive electrical charge, but because electrons orbiting the nucleus have an overall negative charge, an atom with equal numbers of protons and electrons is considered stable.

The properties of an atom vary with the number of electrons and their arrangement in shells around the nucleus. Electrons are organized into distributions of subshells called **electron configurations**. Subshells fill from the inside (closest to the nucleus) to the outside and are lettered starting with "k." The strength of the bond between the nucleus and the electron is called the **binding energy**. The binding energy is stronger for those shells located closer to the nucleus.

The number of electrons in each shell can be determined using the following equation using n for the shell number:

$$2n^2$$

Nature of Electricity

The nature of electricity is based on the atoms of a given material, as objects develop electric charges when their atoms gain or lose electrons. The electrons that are in the furthest shell from an atom's nucleus are the most likely to interact, so they are specially termed **valence electrons**. If the electrons are tightly bound to their atoms, the material is an **insulator** because, like rubber, wood, and glass, the material prevents electrons from flowing freely. However, if the electrons are loosely bound to the atoms, the material is a **conductor** because, like iron and other metals, the electrons can flow freely throughout the material.

It is important to note that opposite charges attract each other, while like charges repel each other. Interestingly, the repulsive force between two electrons is equivalent to the attractive force between an electron and a proton (only in different directions). Coulomb described these repellant and attractive forces between two objects in his namesake law. This electrical **Coulomb force, F,** is determined by multiplying the charges of the two objects, q_1 and q_2, by a constant, k, and dividing by the distance they are from one another squared, r^2.

$$F = \frac{kq_1q_2}{r^2}$$

If the force is negative, then the objects attract each other because q_1 and q_2 are of opposite charges. If the force is positive, then the objects repel each other because q_1 and q_2 are of the same charge.

An electric charge naturally produces an electric field around itself. Electric fields can vary in strength and magnitude depending on the type of charge (positive or negative) that generates the field. The nature of electric fields can be tested using a test charge. Mathematically, the magnitude of an electric field (E) can be found using the following equation:

$$E = \frac{F}{q_o}$$

Where F is the force a test charge would undergo, and q_o is the magnitude of the test charge. Electric fields are vector quantities; this means they have both a magnitude and a direction. In the case of electric fields, it is the convention to define the direction of the field vector as the way a positive test charge would move when positioned in the electric field: towards a negative charge and away from other positive charges.

An **electric circuit** is usually comprised of circuit elements joined by a wire or other object that allows an electric charge to move along the path without interruption—this moving electric charge is called an electric **current.** However, constant electric currents may only exist in a complete circuit if there is a voltage difference in the circuit. **Voltage** is literally the distance that a circuit's electrical force could move one electron, but voltage can be visualized as how much energy a certain part of the circuit has available to push around electrons. Electrons will flow from regions of higher voltage to regions of lower voltage, so it is the difference in voltages between two parts of a circuit that makes a current actually flow.

In other words, voltage difference is the difference in potential energy between two places measured in **volts (V),** while a circuit is a closed path through which electrons can flow. Because every atom has positive charges that pull on electrons and resist their flow, most real circuits have a **resistance** level, measured in **ohms,** which is described as the opposition to the flow of electric charge. The amount of current that can flow through a circuit depends on the voltage difference and how well the wire resists the flow of electricity. **Ohm's law** gives us the relationship between voltage (V), current in amperes (I), and resistance in ohms (R).

$$V = I \times R$$

Series Circuits (A) and Parallel Circuits (B)

Practical circuits have numerous loads which can be hooked up "in series" (A) or "in parallel" (B), as shown below.

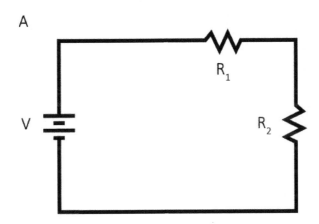

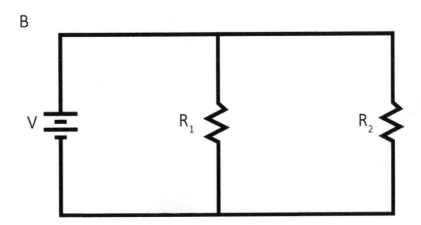

To determine the total voltage requirement for circuits with multiple component loads (in series or in parallel), it is necessary to find the equivalent resistance of the circuits.

Series circuits put resistors in a row or series so that current must flow from one to the other, while **parallel circuits** run resistors in parallel sections so that current can flow through one or the other. In a series circuit like the one in *A*, the voltage drops across each resistor, but the current is the same in all of them. The current must be the same across each resistor, as according to Ampere's law, the electrons in the current must continue flowing throughout the wire and not build up or disappear. In other words, the electrons going into the resistor must all go out so that the "flow in equals flow out."

The current through each resistor is the same, and the total voltage (*V*) equals the drop across R_1 plus the drop across R_2. The equivalent resistance is determined by solving Ohm's law for voltage:

$$V = V_1 + V_2 = IR_1 + IR_2 = I(R_1 + R_2) = IR_{eq}$$

Thus, in a series circuit, the equivalent resistance is equal to the sum of the component resistances, and this relation holds for any number of resistors in a series.

In a parallel circuit like the one in *(B)*, the voltage is the same across each resistor because each is attached directly to the power source and the ground. The electric current is divided between the loads depending on their resistances, since it can flow through either of them, but not both. If the resistance is the same in both loads, then the same amount of current passes through each one. If the resistance is different in each load, then more current passes through the load with the lower resistance, since energy takes the path of least resistance.

The **equivalent resistance (R_{eq})** of the parallel circuit is determined by solving Ohm's law for the current through each resistor, setting it equal to the total current (R_t), and remembering that the voltages are all the same:

$$I_t = \frac{V}{R_{eq}} = \frac{V}{R_1} + \frac{V}{R_2} \quad \textit{or} \quad \frac{1}{R_{eq}} = \frac{1}{R_1} + \frac{1}{R_2} \quad \textit{so} \quad R_{eq} = \frac{1}{\frac{1}{R_1} + \frac{1}{R_2}}$$

In a parallel circuit, the equivalent resistance is equal to one over the sum of the reciprocals of the component resistances.

Magnetism and Electricity

Magnetism can occur naturally in certain types of materials like iron, nickel, and cobalt. If two straight rods are made from iron, they will usually have a naturally negative end (pole) and a positive end (pole). These charged poles react just like any charged item: opposite charges attract and like charges repel. They will attract each other when set up positive to negative, but if one rod is turned around, the two rods will repel each other due to the alignment of negative to negative and positive to positive.

Magnetic fields can also be created and amplified by using an electric current. The force of attraction between two magnetic fields is measured in **Teslas**. The relationship between magnetic forces and electrical forces can be explored by sending an electric current through a stretch of wire, which creates an electromagnetic force around the wire from the charge of the current, as long as the flow of electricity is sustained. This magnetic force can also attract and repel other items with magnetic properties. Depending upon the strength of the current in the wire, a smaller or larger magnetic force can be generated around this wire. As soon as the current is cut off, the magnetic force also stops. When a magnetic field produces an electric current, this is called an **electromagnetic induction**.

Practice Questions

1. Velocity is a measure of which of the following?
    a. Speed with direction
    b. The change in speed over the change in time
    c. Acceleration with direction
    d. All of the above

2. What is the definition of acceleration?
    a. The rate at which an object moves
    b. The rate of change in velocity
    c. Speed in a given direction
    d. The velocity of an object multiplied by its mass

3. Which of the following is NOT one of Newton's three laws of motion?
    a. An object a rest tends to stay at rest, and an object in motion tends to stay in motion
    b. $E = mc^2$
    c. For every action, there is an equal and opposite reaction
    d. $F = ma$

4. For circular motion, what is the name of the actual force pulling toward the axis of rotation?
    a. Centrifugal force
    b. Gravity
    c. Centripetal force
    d. No force is acting

5. The energy of motion is also referred to as what?
    a. Potential energy
    b. Kinetic energy
    c. Electric energy
    d. Electromagnetic energy

6. What is the purpose of a wave?
    a. To carry matter
    b. To transfer energy
    c. To do work
    d. To slow down matter

7. What is the term for when a wave bends?
    a. Refraction
    b. Diffraction
    c. Reflection
    d. Convection

8. Which of the following reside in the nucleus of an atom?
    a. Protons and neutrons
    b. Neutrons and electrons
    c. Electrons and ions
    d. Ions and protons

9. How does electrical energy flow?
   a. From objects with lesser potential energy to objects with greater potential energy
   b. Equally between objects with equal potential energy
   c. From objects with greater potential energy to objects with lesser potential energy
   d. From objects with greater magnetic energy to objects with greater electrical energy

10. Which of the following is true regarding electromagnetism?
    a. Opposite charges attract
    b. Like charges attract
    c. Opposite charge are neutral towards one another
    d. Like charges are neutral towards one another